Healthiest YOU EVER

365 WAYS TO

Lose Weight, Build Strength, Boost Your BMI, Lower Your Blood Pressure, Increase Your Stamina, Improve Your Cholesterol Levels, and **ENERGIZE FROM HEAD TO TOE!**

Meera Lester, Murdoc Khaleghi, MD, Susan Reynolds, and Brett Aved

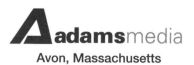

Aadamsmedia

Avon, Massachusetts

Published by
Adams Media, a division of F+W Media, Inc.
57 Littlefield Street, Avon, MA 02322. U.S.A.
www.adamsmedia.com

ISBN 10: 1-4405-3004-1
ISBN 13: 978-1-4405-3004-3
eISBN 10: 1-4405-3116-1
eISBN 13: 978-1-4405-3116-3

Printed in the United States of America.

10 9 8 7 6 5 4 3 2 1

Library of Congress Cataloging-in-Publication Data
is available from the publisher.

This book is intended as general information only, and should not be used to diagnose or treat any health condition. In light of the complex, individual, and specific nature of health problems, this book is not intended to replace professional medical advice. The ideas, procedures, and suggestions in this book are intended to supplement, not replace, the advice of a trained medical professional. Consult your physician before adopting any of the suggestions in this book, as well as about any condition that may require diagnosis or medical attention. The author and publisher disclaim any liability arising directly or indirectly from the use of this book.

Many of the designations used by manufacturers and sellers to distinguish their product are claimed as trademarks. Where those designations appear in this book and Adams Media was aware of a trademark claim, the designations have been printed with initial capital letters.

This book is available at quantity discounts for bulk purchases.
For information, please call 1-800-289-0963.

INTRODUCTION

If you're healthy, you have more wealth than money could ever buy. But are you as healthy as you could be? Even if you're doing a hundred things right—watching your weight, working out a few days a week, eating plenty of fruits and vegetables, limiting food with too much sugar or saturated fat, feeding and challenging your brain, nurturing your spirit as well as your flesh—there's also a lot more you can do. Fortunately, *Healthiest You Ever* is designed to offer you a full year of actionable information in seven categories, one for each day of the week, so you can do something every day to improve your health and fitness. The categories are as follows:

Monday: Diet and Nutrition
Tuesday: Strength
Wednesday: Mental Agility
Thursday: Endurance
Friday: Flexibility
Saturday: Recreation
Sunday: Rest

As you work your way through the book you'll notice that the fitness items progress from the easiest or beginning levels of each activity to the harder, more difficult items. This way, you can start slowly and build toward improved flexibility, increased strength, and bolstered endurance. Some of the suggestions overlap, but each offers a new aspect, a new level, or a new attitude that can lead to progress or a deepening of your practice. The entries on rest include everything from actual sleep to meditation to spiritual renewal. And throughout the book you'll also find a wealth of recreational activities that will bolster your fitness—and your fun!

Together, the 365 entries found within will provide you with a game plan for vastly improving your overall health and fitness. The mere fact that you've picked up this book means that you're someone who takes personal responsibility and who strives to become an ever-better version of yourself. All you need to do is put the plan in motion by picking up the proverbial sword and marching boldly forward—one day at a time. So, hurry up, turn the page, and get started!

"Eighty percent of weight loss comes as a result of wise food choices."

—Fitz Koehler, fitness expert

Keep a Food Diary for at Least a Week

Do you even know how much and when you eat during a typical day? Most people don't. The best way to learn is to keep a food journal for at least a week. Using a notebook, your iPad, your smart phone, your running log, or a calendar (something you can keep a record in), write down everything you eat and when you eat it. Don't cheat! List even the breath mints you chew on during meetings. It's also helpful to note where your eating has taken place—at your desk? in the cafeteria? in front of the TV?—and how you were feeling at the time—super stressed? depressed? tipsy? This will help you identify your eating triggers and whatever bad habits you may have formed regarding eating.

After a full week you'll have a good idea of the what, when, where, and why of your eating patterns. From the brief discussion here, you should be able to see from your food diary where you're making your nutritional no-noes. How often have you skipped breakfast? How often have you eaten high-fat foods like junk food, desserts, and fried food? What are your snacking habits? How many fruits and vegetables do you eat in a typical week? How often do you eat because you're feeling blue or stressed, rather than hungry? Which foods do you gravitate toward to elevate your moods? CARBS

WEEK ONE

"When you first start weight training, don't be surprised if you actually gain weight. This is a normal reaction for many people. The average person starting an exercise program may gain 3 to 5 pounds. If you're among these people, you've successfully gained lean body mass or muscles. Congratulate yourself. You deserve a pat on the back for all your hard work!"

—Shirley S. Archer, fitness professional, Stanford University School of Medicine

Check Your Body Composition

Your body composition refers to the percentage of fat and percentage of fat-free body mass that makes up your total body weight. Fat-free mass, also known as lean-body mass, consists primarily of muscle tissue, bones, and blood, essentially all the rest of your body that is not fat.

Research suggests that the ideal percentage of body fat for men is 15 to 18 percent. For women, the ideal range of body fat is 22 to 25 percent. It's important to remember that these are suggested ranges. Some individuals with a higher percentage of body fat who are regularly active may still be considered at a healthy weight.

When you begin your improvement program, you might want to measure your body composition. This way, you'll have a baseline against which to measure the effectiveness of your program over time. You can see how much muscle mass you have when you get started. Every six weeks or so, you can check to see how much more muscle mass you have developed. If you're a person who is motivated by numbers, this is a concrete way to stay excited about your progress.

"Exercise doesn't make you smarter, but what it does
do is optimize the brain for learning."

—Dr. John J. Ratey, MD, Harvard Medical School

Exercise for Thirty Minutes a Day

Regular exercise is essential if you're looking to preserve your mental acuity. Aerobic exercise helps get the blood coursing through your system, carrying oxygen and glucose to your brain—two substances the brain needs in order to function. Regular exercise can also prod the brain into producing more molecules that help protect and produce the brain's neurons. Though studies are still underway to establish the link between exercise and increased brain neurons, many researchers—including those involved with Alzheimer's disease research—are studying the protective effects of regular physical exercise on the brain's neural paths for transmitting signals.

The U.S. federal guidelines for exercise say that getting at least thirty minutes a day most days a week will help prevent heart disease, osteoporosis, diabetes, obesity, and now, perhaps, Alzheimer's. If you do nothing else, a brisk thirty-minute walk every day will do wonders for your brain health.

IT ALSO KEEPS YOUR BRAIN YOUNG

As you get older, exercise becomes even better for your overall brain health. Neuroscientists have shown that in aging populations (usually those over age sixty-five), sustained, moderate exercise participation enhances learning and memory, improves the function of the neocortex, counteracts age-related and disease-related mental decline, and protects against age-related atrophy in brain areas crucial for thinking and learning. Exercise has been cited by several researchers, including those at UC Irvine, as being the number one factor in sustaining brain health and the ability to make new neurons in an aging brain.

"My attitude is that if you push me towards something that you think is a weakness, then I will turn that perceived weakness into a strength."

—Michael Jordan

Understand the Difference Between Strength and Endurance

Muscular strength and endurance are equally important, and they are closely related in that it requires a certain amount of strength to develop endurance. For example, in order to develop upper body muscular endurance through pushups, you must have the strength to do at least one pushup. The inability to do a pushup is a lack of strength, not a lack of endurance.

For the most part, the same exercises are used to increase muscular strength and endurance. The only difference is the amount of resistance and the number of repetitions one completes in a set. In general, muscular strength is best developed by high resistance (heavy weight) and low repetition (short time period) exercises, while muscular endurance is improved by using less resistance (low weight) and higher repetitions (or a longer time period).

You can have strength without endurance. However, it is nearly impossible to develop muscular endurance without also developing strength. There are weightlifters who can bench press over 500 pounds, as long as they only have to push it up one time. However, some of these lifters are unable to do twenty pushups. So endurance training supplemented with a weight program is beneficial.

"Flexibility falls under the 'use it or lose it' rule. You have to practice consistently, and the one thing people tend to forget is that strength and flexibility go hand in hand."

—Nathan Brown, martial arts instructor

Practice a Variety of Stretches

Exercise books and videos offer differing advice on what stretch to do, how long to hold a stretch, how often you need to stretch, and so on. The answer to all of these questions is different from person to person and every expert will give different advice. What is important is that you make sure to take the time to lengthen your muscles in some way. It helps to know the four types of stretches:

- **Active:** This type of stretching is usually used within the warm-up of a training session. You can take almost any stretch and make it active by moving in and out of the stretch using your breath.
- **Dynamic:** This is another efficient technique within the warm-up. It involves momentum and muscular effort in order to move primary joints that are going to be used during activity. Big shoulder circles, leg swings, hip circles, and standing spinal rotations are all considered dynamic stretches.
- **Passive:** A passive stretch is considered a relaxing, cooling, and calming type of stretch. Passive stretches do not require you to hold your body weight while lengthening a muscle. These are mostly done in the seated or lying down position, and exhaling is emphasized to recruit the relaxation response.
- **Static:** A static stretch is one that has no movement involved but muscles are recruited to hold the position. These exercises are usually, but not always, weight bearing in nature. Holding a High Lunge with your arms over your head, a Downward Facing Dog pose, and a Kneeling Hamstring Stretch are all considered static stretches.

"You can't get rid of it [fat] with exercise alone. You can do the most vigorous exercise and only burn up 300 calories in an hour. If you've got fat on your body, the exercise firms and tones the muscles. But when you use that tape measure, what makes it bigger? It's the fat!"

—Jack LaLanne

Buy Some Hand-Weights and Use Them to Exercise at Home

Sustaining a brisk pace and steady heart rate is not the only important form of exercise. Increasing your strength is important, too. By increasing your muscle mass, not only do you convert the calories of protein into muscle, but your new muscle gets the calories it needs to function, increasing your metabolism.

In fact, more and more research suggests lifting weights may be one of the most efficient forms of losing weight. Not only are calories required to perform the exercise, but calories are also needed to build muscle. In addition, muscle has a higher metabolism than fat, so when you bulk up your muscles, you will have a higher metabolism and burn more calories, even at rest.

START SLOWLY, BUILD STEADILY

Sports stores sell hand-weights or weighted balls that you can buy. Start there and slowly build toward a more intensive weight-lifting program, at which point you might want to join a gym. Start out by lifting 2- or 5-pound weights, and slowly build your ability to do more and more repetitions. You don't have to lift heavy weights for the activity to have an impact.

*"A person who has good thoughts cannot ever be ugly. You can have
a wonky nose and a crooked mouth and a double chin and stick-out
teeth, but if you have good thoughts they will shine out of your face like
sunbeams and you will always look lovely."*

—Roald Dahl

Spend the Day Thinking Happy Thoughts

If you want to find happiness and add years to your life, think happy
thoughts. When you choose positive thoughts over negative ones,
you are more likely to develop an optimistic outlook on life. According to happiness researchers such as Martin E. P. Seligman, director of
the Positive Psychology Center at the University of Pennsylvania, and
Barbara Fredrickson, PhD, professor of psychology at the University
of North Carolina at Chapel Hill, positive people generally have higher
levels of optimism and life satisfaction and live longer. In a BBC News
report, Dr. Seligman was quoted as saying that he believed that "we
have compelling evidence that optimists and pessimists will differ markedly in how long they live." Dr. Fredrickson has counseled that changing your mindset can change your body chemistry. She has stated that
positive feelings literally can open the heart and mind. And there's more
good news. Even if you aren't normally a happy person, thinking happy
thoughts is a skill that can be learned. Work on being open, being an
optimist, choosing to think positive thoughts, and seeing the proverbial
glass half full rather than half empty.

"Although 67 percent of Americans report taking calories into account when making food purchases, nearly nine out of ten have no idea how many they actually need."

—The International Food Information Council Foundation

Figure Out How Many Calories You Burn a Day

Calories provide energy for your body, but your metabolism decides how it's going to use the calories you eat. If you take in more calories than your body requires, your body will generally store the extra calories as fat. Therefore, when you consume more calories than you need over a period of time, you gain weight. If you take in fewer calories than your body requires, or burn calories via exercise, your body will call upon the stores of fat to meet its energy requirements. If you do this over a period of time, you will lose weight.

If you are taking in more calories than your body can metabolize and burn as energy and you want to lose weight, you will have to reduce the amount of calories you take in, increase the number of calories you burn through physical exercise, or most likely do both. It is difficult to maintain your desired weight as you age or lose weight without changing the output side of the metabolism equation; that is, you need to boost your metabolism and increase its efficiency by eating healthfully and by exercising regularly and rigorously.

METABOLISM CALCULATORS

In order to determine your ideal caloric intake, it's crucial to know your metabolic rate, or the rate at which your body burns calories. This number will give you a concrete idea of how many calories you need to maintain your current weight, or how many you need to cut to lose weight. Metabolism calculators are available on many medical websites, such as the following on Webmd .com: *www.webmd.com/diet/healthtool-metabolism-calculator.*

"Running is real and relatively simple . . . but it ain't easy."

—Mark Will-Weber

Add Running to Your Repertoire

Running offers amazing health benefits—and it makes your whole body stronger. Here are some benefits to be gained from running (and you don't have to run five miles a day to start seeing benefits; add ¼ mile every two days and slowly build to one mile twice a week):

- It improves respiration for both resting and activity-related breathing.
- It improves cardiac output and efficiency and makes your heart stronger.
- It improves circulation, flushes arteries, and lowers blood pressure.
- It improves muscular strength and endurance.
- It increases bone density.
- It improves joint flexibility and mobility.
- It improves bowel functioning.
- It improves balance and movement.
- It increases production of endorphins and improves cognition.

So, even if the thought of running leaves you feeling cold, if you're serious about gaining strength and improving your overall health and you don't have any body issues that would preclude running, you should at least give it a try. Start with a slow jog, for short distances, and see if transitioning to running might be easier than you think.

"Strengthening neural systems is not fundamentally different [than strengthening certain muscle groups through physical exercise]. It's basically replacing certain habits of mind with other habits."

—Richard Davidson, PhD

Exercise Your Brain Too!

Numerous studies have shown that people who lead lives with little mental stimulation experience greater cognitive loss as they age. Their memory fails with greater frequency, and they find it increasingly difficult to work puzzles, perform mathematic equations, and do other mental feats that come quite easily to people who "exercise" their brains often. Maintaining mental acuity is like training to be a professional athlete; you need to do something every day that revs up your brain and flexes your gray matter. Treat your brain like a muscle, one that needs a strenuous workout on a regular basis.

RESPECT YOUR ELDERS . . . ELDER BRAIN CELLS, THAT IS

Cells in the lining of our mouth and intestines live for only a few days, and red blood cells live an average of three months. But nerve cells—which generate while you're still floating in your mother's uterus—can live 100 years or longer! It was once thought that nerve cells weren't replaced when they died, but recent studies show that new nerve cells can arise in a few regions of the brain, even in older brains. This increases the importance of supporting and stimulating your brain, not only to improve the longevity of your existing nerve cells, but also for production of new nerve cells. Your brain and body do their jobs by ensuring an ongoing process of cellular detoxification and repair, but it's up to you to provide the nurturance and stimulation required to keep your brain cells awake and alive.

"The five S's of sports training are: Stamina, Speed, Strength, Skill, and Spirit; but the greatest of these is Spirit."

—Ken Doherty

Learn How to Take Your Pulse

To monitor your heart rate during endurance training, you will need to know how to take your pulse—both to measure your resting heart rate and your working out heart rate. To measure your exercise heart rate, the preferred locations are either at your neck (the carotid pulse) or at your wrist (the radial pulse). Choose the location that works best for you.

Here's a handy method to locate your carotid pulse at your neck. Take your first two fingertips and place them outside of your eye on your temple. Slide your fingertips down from the middle of your temple to the side of your neck. You should start to feel the pulse. Be sure not to press on your pulse or to massage your neck. Use a gentle touch.

To find your radial pulse at your wrist, place your wrist palm facing up in the palm of your other hand. Wrap your fingers around your wrist. You should feel the pulse in the area between the bone and the tendons.

Once you locate your pulse, follow these simple steps to count. Start counting immediately. For your exercise pulse, take a ten-second count. Multiply that number by six for your one-minute heart rate. If you're taking your resting heart rate first thing in the morning, count for a full one minute. A one-minute count isn't recommended for your exercise heart rate as your pulse will slow down from the time you start taking the count to when you finish. Be sure to keep your legs moving while taking your exercise heart rate. You can either walk or march in place.

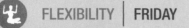

"Blessed are the flexible, for they shall not be bent out of shape."

—Author Unknown

Warm Up Before You Stretch for Improved Flexibility

Stretching is perhaps *the* most important thing you can do to improve your flexibility. However, stretching a muscle without first warming it up will not result in significant long-term improvements in flexibility—and it could lead to damage. If you really want to increase your flexibility, you'll need to stretch when your muscles are warm and elastic. And, if you want to target specific areas for improvement in flexibility, you will need to develop a flexibility-training program, about which we'll have a lot to suggest throughout this book.

In fact, to improve your overall flexibility, the ideal time to stretch a muscle is after you've exercised and raised your body's temperature. When you're weight training, for example, this would be right after you've performed your strength-training set for that particular muscle group. Your muscles are warm and primed. Some people prefer to save their stretching for their final cool down after they're finished with their entire exercise program, which works well if you're short on time.

WORK STRETCHING INTO YOUR WORKOUT

Try stretching throughout a workout after each muscle group has been challenged. At the end of your complete program, take about ten to fifteen additional minutes for a full-body stretch. This is a great time to simply relax, tune in to your body, and reap the rewards of your gym efforts. Whichever way you prefer, the bottom line is that stretching is good for you and should be incorporated into your workout.

"We estimate that we get a quarter of a million people.
Shoppers come in from all over the country, even internationally."

—Scott Sandman on the "World's Longest Yard Sale" spanning 450 miles

Clean House, Free Up Space, and Donate to Local Charities

Having a yard sale is a great way to get a workout, free up space, and earn money you can donate. Advertise that your yard sale will donate all proceeds to charity, and you'll soon have enthusiastic buyers eager to help you help others. Here are a few ideas for donating whatever is left over from the yard sale:

- Donate to charitable consignment shops. Some communities have thrift stores to benefit the Cancer Society or Catholic Charities or mental health centers for kids. There are also battered women's shelters that need many items, from household goods to clothing for women who are trying to put their lives back together.
- Recycle using Freecycle.com. If there isn't one where you live, start a Freecycle branch. The Freecycle network is a virtual organization of and for people who wish to recycle rather than throw stuff into landfills. Find items you need and get them free or post items that you want to give away at *www.freecycle.com*.
- Recycle nonrecyclable materials. Companies like TerraCycle (*www.terracycle.net*) are taking packaging materials from products like energy bars and drink pouches and making them into new products, from tote bags to homework folders. You can mail in your used materials or drop them off at a local center.

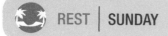

"The air was fragrant with a thousand trodden aromatic herbs,
with fields of lavender, and with the brightest roses blushing
in tufts all over the meadows. . . ."

—William Cullen Bryant

Set Out a Bowl of Freshly Crushed Lavender

Whenever you have a bad day, feel exasperated, and struggle to get out of a foul mood, use some lavender to restore your serenity. Lavender is one of aromatherapy's most popular scents. Scents like lavender, citrus, rose, and sandalwood can trigger particular memories or experiences associated with them. That's because your olfactory nerve carries the scent straight to your brain. Use freshly crushed flowers set out in bowl, insert some reeds in a diffuser pot with lavender essential oil, light some lavender-scented candles, or put out some sachets of dried lavender. Allow the scent to lift your mood and remember that you never have to live a bad day over again.

"When in doubt, check your diet. Your diet is absolutely key when you're having issues losing fat. Try to really watch your carbs at night (after 6 P.M.). Try to stick with lean protein and veggies later in the day and you should see a great improvement in your physique."

—Kris Bierek, founder of Shape-fit.com

Push Past Weight-Loss Plateaus

Ever wonder why heavier people seem to lose weight faster? Surprisingly, the more weight you carry, the faster your metabolism. Having to carry around the extra weight forces your metabolism to fire up. Sounds good, but this creates unwelcome weight-loss plateaus. As you lose weight, your body doesn't need to work as hard to metabolize food into energy, so it slows down the process. Unfortunately, the only way to combat this plateau is to stick with the diet (and gradually lower caloric intake) and increase the amount and/or intensity of your workouts. The slimmer you become, the fewer calories you'll need to maintain good health—deal with it.

Increasing the intensity of workouts is a great way to push past the plateaus, but there are also two very doable (no excuses!) tactics for pushing past a weight-loss plateau that anyone can adopt:

- **Add a Brisk Morning Walk.** The one time when simple aerobic exercise can really boost your metabolism is in the morning. When you first wake up, your liver has burned through your carbohydrate stores, and light aerobic exercise can jump-start the fat-burning enzymes in your liver.
- **Eat More Vegetables.** Fiber is a non-digestible carbohydrate, but the body tries hard to break it down anyway, using up energy—and boosting metabolism in the process. Plus, vegetables are low in calories, yet high in nutrients, which provides a huge boon for your weight loss efforts.

WEEK THREE

"I was pushed by myself because I have my own rule, and that is that every day I run faster and try harder."

—William Sigei

Commit to Running a Few Days a Week

First, let go of preconceived ideas about fitness and running. Acknowledge and release old negative attitudes. Maybe you think you will never enjoy running. Think instead about the benefits it provides: new friends, improved energy, a better mood, and healthier lifestyle. Keep in mind that you don't start running by doing a marathon. Set short workouts as a goal, and be proud of what you accomplish. Learn by taking small steps, and your relationship with running (or walking/running) will become a lifelong love affair.

Think of your running time as an investment in your health that yields invaluable returns. By committing only one half-hour a day (that's less than 2 percent of your whole day!), you can reap the rewards. You—not other market conditions—control this investment. Regular running is vital to achieving optimal health while also helping to protect you from many preventable diseases. Running costs can be less expensive than what you pay for most life insurance policies, and you realize the benefits while you are still alive.

And if running is too stressful, or something you're not quite ready to tackle on a regular basis, go powerwalking instead. The point is to move your behind at a rapid clip. Start at whatever level you feel confident about, but start.

GET YOUR MINDSET ON

Take a minute to write down five reasons why you want to get fit through incorporating running in your life. You may be surprised by your reasons, which in turn might change over time. Review your answers in one month, then two, to see your progress.

"Most men pursue pleasure with such breathless haste that they hurry past it."

—Soren Kierkegaard

Do Something Fun to Relieve Stress

Chronic stress kills . . . *literally.* It's been widely shown to have disastrous physical effects, but did you know that chronic stress also diverts energy from your brain (fogs up your mind), shrinks your hippocampus (slows memory and learning), compromises neurotransmitters (limiting joy *and* plasticity), and even emits toxins that attack your brain? Forget zombies, stress eats your brain. Make it a priority to relax. Doing things that are physically and mentally stimulating and energizing is fine, but they also have to be relaxing—with an emphasis on fun.

Here's a list of suggestions for activities that will immediately stimulate your pleasure centers:

- A romantic dinner date in your favorite Italian restaurant
- Soaking in a tub filled with luxurious bath salts
- A hot stone massage at your favorite spa
- A long walk through the woods near your house
- Taking your dogs to the beach for the day
- Sitting by the fire while reading a juicy novel
- Stockpiling your cupboard with fresh spices
- Buying new sheets in your favorite color
- Fooling around under the sheets with your partner.

"No one ever drowned in sweat."

—Dan Gable

Determine Your Target Heart Rate Using the Karvonen Formula

If you're ready for endurance training, it's likely that you've been conditioning through exercise for a while. If so, you may be one of the lucky ones—your physiological age may be younger than your biological age. If you think you fall into that category, rather than using the usual age formula for calculating your target heart rate zone, you may want to use the Karvonen Formula. The Karvonen Formula, also known as the heart rate reserve method, provides a more personalized estimate of your target heart rate zone. Here's how:

1. Subtract your age from 220. This is your maximum heart rate.
2. Subtract your resting heart rate (which you've determined by taking your resting pulse in Week Two) from your maximum heart rate. This number is referred to as your heart rate reserve.
3. Multiply your heart rate reserve by 60 percent.
4. Take this number and add your resting heart rate. This number is the lower end of your target training zone.
5. Take your heart rate reserve and multiply by 80 percent.
6. Take this number and add your resting heart rate. This number is the upper end of your target training zone.

Again, if you are just beginning endurance training, don't aim for the upper end out of the gate. Instead, start low and work your way to the upper end of your target training zone.

"Experts agree that stretching should be part of an overall exercise program to improve health."

—Shirley S. Archer, fitness professional, Stanford School of Medicine

Practice Safe Stretch

Safe technique is essential when stretching. For starters, pay attention to your alignment. Avoid excessive arching of the back. Keep your abdominal muscles active with a feeling of tone to provide support for your lower back.

Your stretching movements should be slow and controlled. Do not use force. When you execute the movement, proceed gently to the extent of your active range of motion. This is the largest possible movement you can achieve without feelings of strain. As you hold the stretch and breathe, your muscles will relax and lengthen. Allow the muscle to release into the stretch and increase the size of your stretch as your muscles permit. Always let your muscles lead the stretch. Never force your muscles into a longer position.

Avoid forced or rapid movements as they can trigger a stretch reflex. A stretch reflex is your body's natural way of protecting you from overly lengthening a muscle and harming the integrity of a joint. If you suddenly force a muscle to lengthen, the stretch reflex will trigger a contraction.

Hold your stretches for fifteen to thirty seconds. According to some research studies, it's more beneficial to stretch multiple times rather than to hold one long stretch for an excessive period of time. For example, in one study, three twenty-second stretches and two thirty-second stretches achieved greater changes in hamstring flexibility than one sixty-second stretch. Across studies, stretches of longer than thirty seconds in duration have not been shown to be more effective in increasing flexibility. What we do know is that experts agree that flexibility is complex and affected by joint mechanics, muscle and connective tissue, and neuromuscular factors—and that static stretching is effective with the least amount of risk.

"It is not the handling of difficult hands that makes the winning player. There aren't enough of them. It is the ability to avoid messing up the easy ones."

—Alan Sontag

Play Bridge (or Poker) with Three Friends Once a Week

There's a reason little old ladies love to play bridge, and it's a good reason—it keeps their memories sharp, and it allows plenty of time for hanging out with people whose company they enjoy. Even gossiping requires and stimulates memory retention. Plus, happiness experts have established that a strong support network is vital to higher life satisfaction levels. Humans were made for loving others. It is from our relationships with spouses, lovers, and friends that we derive meaning and happiness. Having a group of friends to do things with on a regular basis is a path to happiness. So get the cards, call up three friends, and start having some fun playing bridge or another card game.

PEOPLE DO NEED PEOPLE

Your brain "knows" it needs other people and responds by releasing internal opiates—endorphins—that create that lovely feeling we feel when near someone we love and trust. Studies have consistently shown that feeling close, connected, loved, and supported improves your health and overall sense of well-being. Some studies have reported a lowered incidence of anxiety, depression, suicide, illnesses, high blood pressure, heart disease, and even cancer.

"Massage therapists are trained to knead and manipulate the muscles and connective tissue in the body to help the body find its equilibrium after exercise."

—Melissa Roberts, theologian and stress management specialist

Get a Swedish Massage

This common form of massage involves a massage therapist applying oil to the body and certain types of massage strokes—namely, effleurage (gliding), petrissage (kneading), friction (rubbing), and tapotement (tapping)—to increase circulation in muscles and connective tissue, help the body to flush out waste products, and heal injuries. Swedish massage induces a feeling of deep relaxation and increases range of motion. Some Swedish massage therapists also use hydrotherapy, or massage through soaking, steaming, or applying jets of water to the body.

NEED SOMETHING STRONGER: TRY ROLFING

Rolfing is a deep massage designed to restructure the body's muscles and connective tissue to promote better alignment. If you like your massages hard, this one's for you. Some people claim that the deep tissue massage actually releases deeply buried emotions and that emotional outbursts are common during the course of the ten-session program. So if you've got some releasing to do—and who doesn't?—find yourself a rolfing therapist and let it all out.

"Despite all of the amazing medicines and treatments we have, cardiovascular disease is still the number one cause of death and illness in our society."

—Laurence S. Sperling, MD

Keep Track of Your Cholesterol Numbers

Anyone over thirty—or anyone who eats a high-fat diet—should know their cholesterol levels. If you don't, ask your doctor for a total lipoprotein profile so that you are aware not only of your total cholesterol but of each component as well. You may have a total cholesterol level that is desirable, but that doesn't mean your HDL (high-density lipoprotein or "good" cholesterol) and LDL (low-density lipoprotein or "bad" cholesterol) levels are in line. Your total cholesterol level will fall into one of three categories:

1. **Desirable:** less than 200 mg/dL
2. **Borderline high risk:** 200–239 mg/dL
3. **High risk:** 240 mg/dL and over

If you fall within the high-risk range, you have at least twice the risk of heart disease as someone in the desirable range. If you have a cholesterol reading over 240 mg/dL or you have risk factors such as heart disease along with cholesterol readings over 200 mg/dL, your doctor will probably prescribe a cholesterol-lowering medication in combination with a healthy low-fat diet and exercise. You can lower your negative cholesterol and improve your positive cholesterol levels significantly through improved nutrition and exercise. If you want to live a long life, with a healthy heart, arm yourself with knowledge and take control of your cholesterol levels.

"Ability is what you are capable of doing. Motivation determines what you do. Attitude determines how well you do it."

—Lou Holtz

Consider Joining a Gym to Bolster Your Workouts

Lifting weights is one of the most efficient forms of building muscle. While there are still some gyms that cater to the intense bodybuilder, most gyms, like the YMCA and many commercial health clubs, serve the regular person who just wants to be healthier and get in shape. Joining a gym means having access to multiple machines, as well as free weights, or weights not attached to a machine. The best way to start is on gym machines, most of which show the exercise you can do right on them, so you can simply follow the instructions. If you still feel uncomfortable, work with a personal trainer who can show you some basic exercises. Once you get comfortable on machines, you can try "hybrid" machines, or machines where the resistance used is free weights. While you are getting comfortable on these machines, pay attention to those around you. Other people can serve as great instructors, simply by watching.

Eventually, you may feel comfortable using totally free weights, including barbells and dumbbells. The benefit of these weights is that since they are free, you must use stabilizing "accessory" muscles that you may not need to use with machines. Start with light weights and work your way up. When lifting heavier weights, use a spotter, a person who can grab the weight if you feel unable to lift it, for safety reasons. The last thing you want is for a dropped weight to scare you away from this invaluable activity.

"I am always doing that which I cannot do, in order that I may learn how to do it."

—Pablo Picasso

Stimulate Your Brain by Giving It Novel Experiences

Giving your brain new (novel) experiences helps it to form new neuronal pathways, i.e., whatever you focus on will generate activity and growth in the areas of your brain that are required for that activity, particularly if it's something you've never done before. The more you do something, the more synapses your brain fires and creates. Novelty is great because it will stimulate synapses that have lain dormant or create entirely new ones, because your brain is trying to adapt to process and understand whatever it is that you deem important. Here are some ideas:

- If you're athletic, try something that will flex your cerebellum more than your biceps, something requiring precise movement and muscle control, like dancing.
- If you're an obsessive reader, try learning table tennis (which is supposed to be one of the best physical activities for your brain because it involves anticipation, memory, analysis, and physical coordination, all at a very rapid pace).
- If you never go more than thirty miles from home, plan a 100-mile trip, mapping out back roads that will lead you somewhere exciting (using GPS is cheating!).
- Learn to read music and play a musical instrument. Reading music and playing an instrument has consistently been shown to stimulate your brain in ways that few other activities can. If you're already a musician, take up sculpting or fly-fishing.
- Learn a foreign language, and that means learning to *speak* a foreign language. Join a club that requires you to only speak in the new language—good for your brain and fun!

*"I'm the walkingest girl around. I like to work at it—
really get my heart pounding."*

—Amy Yasbeck

Measure Your Endurance: Take a Walking Test

All you need is a stopwatch or regular watch and your walking shoes,
and then here's what you do:

- Go to a local indoor or outdoor track where you can measure how
  far you walk. If you don't know the exact distance, that's okay. You
  can measure your progress in terms of laps.
- Click the stopwatch or note the time on your watch and begin
  walking. If you don't use a stopwatch, it helps to start at an easily
  remembered point, such as on the hour, quarter hour, or half hour.
  Walk comfortably for ten minutes. If you are not used to walking
  vigorously, do not push yourself. Simply walk at a comfortable
  pace.
- At the end of ten minutes, notice how many laps you have walked.
  Note it down for future reference.

If you want to increase the time of the test, that is okay. Another
way to perform this measurement is to go by distance rather than time.
Rather than walking for ten minutes, you can choose to walk four laps
or you can walk one mile. Whatever method you choose is fine. Be cautious not to push yourself too hard if you are new to exercise.

You can also check your heart rate at the end of the walk. Keep
your feet moving and take your pulse (see Week Two). After one minute
has passed, repeat taking your pulse. Note down both figures. As you
improve you may see reductions in your overall heart rate as well as a
more rapid recovery rate after one minute.

Once you have these numbers, you can use them as a measurement
of your progress as you work toward building endurance.

"You should include flexibility exercises a minimum of two to three days a week in an overall fitness program sufficient to develop and maintain range of motion. These exercises should stretch the major muscle groups."

—The American College of Sports Medicine

Follow the Rules of Static Stretches

Yes, there are rules for static stretches, and following them will benefit your quest for flexibility. Familiarize yourself with the list and get into the habit of following the rules when stretching for flexibility. The rules are:

- Move slowly to the edge of your active range of motion.
- Concentrate on the muscle being stretched.
- Exhale, relax, and allow your muscle to release gradually.
- Inhale, check your alignment.
- Exhale, relax, and continue to lengthen.
- Start with a fifteen-second stretch, work up to twenty or thirty seconds.
- Always move deliberately, with control.
- Increase the stretch as the muscle releases, always working the edge of tension.
- Always feel the stretch in the belly or the central area of the muscle.
- If you feel any pain or tightness in your joint, ease up on the stretch. Pain in your joints means you are stretching too hard.
- Stretch during and at the end of every weight training session.
- Do NOT bounce.
- Do NOT move quickly.
- NEVER apply force.
- Do NOT lock your joints.
- Do NOT go beyond a joint's natural range of motion or hyperextend your joints.

"I don't know if it's just me or everyone, but the whole vibe with skiing is not so much thriving on competition against others as it is against myself and the clock."

—Picabo Street

Go Cross-Country Skiing

During those winter months when running may not be an option, why not break out the cross-country skis? A 150-pound person can burn up to 900 calories per hour as she strengthens the muscles in her shoulders, back, chest, abdomen, buttocks, and legs using the kick and glide technique. If you're looking forward to starting a cross-country routine, we recommend preparing with exercises that work the upper- and lower-body muscle groups such as cycling, walking, swimming, and rowing.

NO SNOW DAYS

As cross-country skiing requires snow, participating in sports or activities that will bolster your skills can make the months between snowfalls productive. Some popular cross-training activities that will improve your cross-country skiing include:

- Cycling (outdoor or stationary)
- Hiking
- Rock climbing
- Inline skating
- Elliptical trainer
- Stair machine
- Nordic Trak (ski machine)

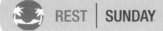

"While making this portage I saw many splendid specimens of the great purple fringed orchis, three feet high. It is remarkable that such delicate flowers should here adorn these wilderness paths."

—Henry David Thoreau

Refresh Yourself in a Scented Bath Amid Orchids

You don't need a reason to indulge in some sensual pleasure. Fill your bathroom with blooming orchids for a super sensual feast for the eyes. Orchids such as oncidiums, cymbidiums, dendrobiums, and paphiopedilums are known for their lush and colorful blooms that can last for weeks. All they need is a little light, warmth, and moisture (bathrooms are perfect places for them). Stick them in antique urns, glazed pottery, or terra-cotta pots. Group them along the window sill, on jardinière shelves, or around a Victorian plant stand. Put on some music. Draw a bath. Drop in your favorite scented oil and a few exquisite orchid blooms. On a bathtub tray or a small table nearby, place a flute filled with sparkling apple cider or champagne, a chocolate truffle, a scented candle, and even a book that inspires you. Take your time, luxuriate, and let the cares and concerns of your day float way. Permit your mind to fill with peaceful, joyful thoughts. When you step out of the bath and back into your world, you will feel renewed and ready to meet whatever challenges may be coming your way.

"Your body is the baggage you must carry through life.
The more excess the baggage, the shorter the trip."

—Arnold H. Glasgow

Lose Belly Fat

In a study of Kaiser Permanente patients in Northern California, middle-aged people with excess visceral fat—more commonly known as belly fat—were nearly three times more likely to suffer from dementia in their seventies and eighties than people with little to no belly fat. The researchers found these people have a much higher risk of having that visceral fat surrounding internal organs deep in their abdominal cavity. Doctors theorize that this fat may release toxins associated with atherosclerosis or the buildup of plaque in the brain that is frequently present in those afflicted with Alzheimer's. The study identified people who were 30 pounds or more overweight who had developed belly fat in their forties as 3.6 times more likely to develop dementia. They reported that the risk for a man with belly fat goes up when his waist exceeds 40 inches; for a woman, it's 35 inches. Doctors recommend a combination of weight training and aerobic exercise that targets the whole body (not just the abdominals), a low-fat diet, and minimal sugar. Surprisingly, recent research has suggested that including dairy products and getting plenty of sleep may help when it comes to battling belly fat.

WEEK FIVE

"Water provides 12 times the resistance of air, so as you walk, you're really strengthening and building muscle."

—Vennie Jones, aquatic fitness coordinator

Warm Up by Taking a Walk in Shallow Water

A great way to warm up your muscles before a weight-lifting workout is to take a walk in shallow water, shallow meaning no more than chest deep. Once in the water, swing your arms freely as if walking on land. This will help your balance and loosen up your back muscles.

Breathe naturally. Concentrate on maintaining good posture with your shoulders relaxed and above your hips and abdominals engaged. Avoid leaning forward excessively. Make sure the opposite arm and leg are moving forward.

Variations to bolster the warm-up:

- (harder) Hold hands out of the water.
- (harder) Walk with elbows in and arms extended outward to increase resistance, while maintaining neutral spine.
- (harder) Increase speed of walking.

Other warm-up ideas include jogging, hopping, traveling lunges, jumping jacks, knee lifts, kicks, rocking, cross-country skiing, bounding, skipping, or backward traveling moves.

"It's cool to be geeky, and sports don't get much geekier than Ping-Pong."

—Susan Sarandon, actress and co-owner of SPiN Gallactic, a Ping-Pong club in New York

Exercise Multiple Areas of Your Brain by Playing Table Tennis

Daniel G. Amen, MD, author of *Making a Good Brain Great*, is a major enthusiast of table tennis, calling it "the best brain sport ever": "It is highly aerobic, uses both the upper and lower body, is great for hand-eye coordination and reflexes, and causes you to use many different areas of the brain at once as you are tracking the ball, planning shots and strategies, and figuring out spins. It is like aerobic chess." He also noted that it is the second most popular organized sport in the world, and has been an Olympic sport since 1988.

Popularly known as Ping-Pong, table tennis requires amazing reflexes, practiced technique, and chess-like strategy. Because the volleys come fast and furious, your brain and muscles have to communicate and respond with lightning speed. Advanced players soon learn to conceal their return's directionality and to add spins that make the game even more challenging. "Everybody I meet either knows somebody or they themselves were at one point a terrific Ping-Pong player," reported Marty Reisman, the 1958 and 1960 United States Open table tennis champion. "Only a small group is cognizant of the extreme skill required to play the game."

"The body's capacity and the soul's capacity, the body's speed and the soul's speed, go together. Running and physical fitness help us both in our inner life of aspiration and in our outer life of activity."

—Sri Chinmoy, international spiritual leader, artist, and activist

Amp Up Your Running Program

Running is one of the best aerobic exercises you can do. Aerobic exercise does for the body what no other activity can because of a crucial process: the utilization of oxygen. You take in oxygen all the time just by breathing, of course. But when you run, you take in greater amounts of oxygen, and it is delivered more deeply into the body because the heart, lungs, and muscles are working harder. Circulation increases and with it, oxygen delivery. This is beneficial for your body and makes you feel good. But even more important for building endurance and increasing stamina, you need a strong focus on aerobic exercises—and running is king.

The body loves regular bouts of oxygen-rich running and like a welcome houseguest makes accommodations for this. The body actually craves a higher aerobic level. The accommodations are the training benefits that improve the working of the body not only during exercise but also while at rest. Plus, when you run, you use one of the body's major tools: its muscles. Running helps to keep your muscles functional and strong, which is essential to endurance.

Ask your doctor if you're healthy enough to amp up your running program. You may want to consult a specialist, too, like an orthopedist or someone who handles sports injuries. You may need to prepare your body first before you begin hard running two or three times a week, particularly as you increase frequency or intensity.

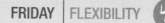

"As you inhale think of lengthening and creating space, and with the exhale think about moving into that space and deepening the stretch."

—Jeff Levine, Krav Maga instructor

Breathe Properly When You Stretch Your Muscles

Controlling your breathing enables you to control other functions of your body, such as heart rate, blood pressure, and respiration. Additionally, conscious deep breathing generates more oxygen for the body and keeps vital lung capacity from decreasing. This can be helpful for cardiovascular activity because it allows more oxygen into the lungs with each breath.

Taking the time to breathe deeply helps to improve your posture and can keep your body from becoming tight and tense. When your body becomes tight and tense, it is very hard to get muscles to lengthen and become more flexible. This is one of the reasons why it is very important to breathe deeply when you are practicing your stretch routine. Through your breath you can stimulate a part of the nervous system that activates the relaxation response. Once you are able to relax you will sleep better, recover from exercise faster, get better from illness faster, and deal with the stresses of life more efficiently.

The best way to use your breath when you are working on a stretch is to inhale as you come up out of the stretch just slightly, then exhale as you move back into the stretch, maybe a little bit further on each sequential breath. Remember: Do not force any stretch. If you use your breath appropriately it will help you relax more into the stretch. Forcing a stretch will make the muscle you are trying to stretch contract and will limit your range of motion. Another way to think of proper breathing is as you inhale you lengthen, as you exhale you deepen the stretch.

"I haven't had sex in eight months.
To be honest, I now prefer to go bowling."

—Lil' Kim

Join a Bowling League

You might not know that the ancient Egyptians enjoyed a good game of bowling. Of course, their balls were stone and players at opposite ends of the lane threw their balls (a big one and a smaller one) at the same time. Today many bowling leagues are looking for a few good participants. Of course, you can bowl alone if that makes you happy, but many people believe that bowling is a game best enjoyed in the company of family or friends. Getting out for a few hours of bowling is good for shifting the constant pressures of home and work and decreasing stress levels while strengthening your friendships by engaging in pleasurable activities with your bowling partners.

While bowling is not the most aerobic of sports, it will get you moving, and something is better than nothing. By signing up for a league, you'll be responsible for showing up for league play every week and expected to do your best. Plus you'll likely burn 219 calories an hour that you might not otherwise have burned.

"Cooking is like love. It should be entered into with abandon or not at all."

—Harriet Van Horne

Cook Your Favorite Dish for Yourself

Cook up something spectacular such as the comfort food of your childhood, an exotic creation you first tasted on your honeymoon, or even a savory palate-pleaser you learned to cook when you were dating that foreign guy or girl. If you are a working parent, then it's unlikely you ever cook just to please yourself. So once in a while, cook what you want to eat instead of only what the kids will eat. They can nibble on pizza, ordered in, while you happily savor every bite of that Moroccan tangine chicken, New England crab cakes, Midwestern meatloaf, Southern fried chicken, or other favorite. You know how happy you feel eating your favorite food. That's why it's your favorite.

"In only thirty days of eating nothing but McDonald's I gained twenty-four and a half pounds, my liver turned to fat and my cholesterol shot up sixty-five points. I nearly doubled my risk of coronary heart disease, making myself twice as likely to have heart failure."

—Morgan Spurlock, *Super Size Me*

Readjust Your Portion Control Meter

Ever since we entered the super size era, Americans have grown much fatter—and our ability to judge what constitutes a healthy portion of food has been skewed. To follow a healthy diet, you don't need to weigh and measure all of your food each day, but you do need to understand that portion size counts and that you may need to readjust your visual image of desirable portions in each food group. Portion sizes are meant as general guidelines and vary according to your sex and age, but for healthy adults, the aim is to come close to the recommended serving sizes, on average, over several days. Use these visual comparisons to help estimate your portion sizes:

- A 3-ounce portion of cooked meat, poultry, or fish is about the size of a deck of playing cards.
- A medium potato is about the size of a computer mouse.
- A cup of rice or pasta is about the size of a fist or a tennis ball.
- A cup of fruit or a medium apple or orange is the size of a baseball.
- A half-cup of chopped vegetables is about the size of three regular ice cubes.
- A 3-ounce portion of grilled fish is the size of your checkbook.
- A 1-ounce piece of cheese is the size of four dice.
- A teaspoon of peanut butter equals one die; 2 tablespoons is about the size of a golf ball.
- An ounce of snack foods—pretzels, etc.—equals a large handful.
- A thumb tip equals 1 teaspoon; 3 thumb tips equal 1 tablespoon; and a whole thumb equals 1 ounce.

"There is no point in being alive if you cannot do the deadlift."

—Jon Pall Sigmarsson

Lift Weights

Weight lifting is an important part of any fitness routine for adults. It builds bone mass and can reverse osteoporosis. It increases muscle tone and helps your body to burn more calories because the more muscle you have, the more calories you burn during the aerobic portion of your workout. Stronger muscles means everyday efforts, from lifting grocery bags and small children to carrying that box of office supplies into the supply room, are easier. You'll feel better, your posture will improve, and your body will look firmer and shapelier.

Lift weights no more than every other day (or every day, but alternating which muscles you work). To find a good plan, talk to your health club trainer, find a good book on weight lifting that addresses your personal goals (toning or building), or subscribe to a magazine, such as *Shape*, that keeps track of the latest news and research on weight lifting and provides different routines with detailed explanations on technique and benefits.

Start with lighter weights and progress to heavier weights as your strength grows.

*"Meditation brings wisdom; lack of meditation leaves ignorance.
Know well what leads you forward and what holds you back,
and choose the path that leads to wisdom."*

—Buddha

Learn to Meditate

In the late 1960s, Harvard cardiologist Herbert Benson, MD, discovered that relaxation methods caused both psychological and physiological changes that served to counterbalance the body's response to "fight or flight." He called this the "relaxation response." Benson's tests showed that people who simply sat quietly with their minds focused on a single word, idea, or thought could markedly change their physiology, decreasing metabolism, slowing heart and respiratory rates, and exhibiting brain waves of the alpha-theta pattern. Benson showed that the relaxation response, no matter how it was achieved, caused bodily transformations: Heart rate, breathing rate, muscle tension, and oxygen consumption fall below resting levels; blood pressure can decrease; and the waking brain shifts into the slower patterns associated with reverie and daydreaming. These slightly altered states of consciousness promote healing in the same way sleep does. Meditation also works to train the mind to avoid negative patterns and thought processes, vicious circles of failure, low self-esteem, and even the perception of chronic pain as an intensely negative experience. The brain is a complex and amazing organ, and meditation can teach you to harness your mind's power, integrate your mind and body, and feed your hungry spirit. Meditation comes in many forms, including sitting meditation, walking meditation, mindfulness meditation, yoga meditation, mantra meditation, mandala meditation, visualization, and even prayer.

"In all our involvement with elite athletes now, we don't do this kind of static stretching anymore . . . [the best science suggests that an ideal preworkout routine] consists of a very easy warm-up, followed by a gradual increase in intensity and then dynamic stretching."

—Ross Tucker, PhD, *The Runner's Body*

Warm Up Before You Workout . . . Stretch *after* Your Workout

A major misconception about working out is that you must stretch beforehand. In fact, the opposite is the case: You should stretch *after* a workout. If you want to loosen up or warm up your muscles before your run, for example, jog or walk for five to ten minutes and then stretch. With all intensive workouts, the best thing to do is to start very slowly, then ease into a training pace five to ten minutes later.

While it's not good to stretch a cold muscle, it's very important to remember to stretch after a workout, particularly if it's an intensive workout. A workout isn't over until, as part of your cool-down period, you stretch thoroughly. Stretching thirty or forty minutes later after your muscles have cooled down actually increases your chances of causing injury, whereas stretching immediately after a long or fast-paced workout can help alleviate soreness later. Successful runners consider the stretching period after the run as important as the run itself.

In short, stretch gently and slowly while your muscles are still warm. One final rule: No bouncing when you stretch. That is called ballistic stretching, and it can cause injuries!

"Muscle mass is not only metabolically more active than fat, it's also denser. That means that pound for pound, muscle takes up less space on your body than fat. And, with respect to mass, muscle weighs more than fat."

—Shirley S. Archer, fitness professional, Stanford University School of Medicine

Become a Long, Lean, Metabolism-Boosting Machine

Exercise keeps your body and all of your parts working efficiently. When your heart is fit, it beats more strongly but uses less energy to keep pumping. When your muscles are fit, they can lift more and work longer without feeling stress or getting hurt. When your entire body is fit, you burn more calories, sleep better at night, and have a stronger immune system and higher metabolic rate. When you exercise regularly and effectively, your body is lean, sleek, and capable. You'll need to do thirty minutes of moderate activity daily (which can be broken up into ten-minute sessions) to stay healthy, and three or four high-intensity workouts each week to stay truly fit. The more you exercise, the more calories you burn, and the stronger your heart and muscles are.

UP THE AMOUNT OF GENERAL EXERCISE YOU GET DAILY

General exercise includes any activity that requires the use of muscles, such as walking around the block, doing housework or yard work, and taking the stairs rather than the elevator. A thirty-minute walk can make a significant difference, as will any other activities that involve total body movement—and we don't mean moving your thumb while playing video games or moving your arms while knitting. Move your body to boost your metabolism and to vastly improve your overall health.

"According to surveys, only 40 percent of adults meet the minimum activity recommendation to provide health benefits of thirty minutes on most days of the week."

—Murdoc Khaleghi, MD

Make Sure You Achieve Moderate Activity

Research shows that activity can come in a variety of ways and still provide health benefits. The good news is that with so many activities to choose from, you are likely to find something that you enjoy and are able to incorporate into your life on a regular basis. The following are examples of moderate amounts of physical activity:

EXAMPLES OF MODERATE AMOUNTS OF ACTIVITIES	
Types of Activity	Length of Time
Playing volleyball	45 minutes
Playing touch football	30–45 minutes
Walking 1¾ miles	35 minutes (20-minute mile, or pace of 3 miles/hour)
Basketball (shooting baskets)	30 minutes
Bicycling 5 miles	30 minutes
Walking 2 miles	30 minutes (15-minute mile, or pace of 4 miles/hour)
Swimming laps	20 minutes

You can also perform some activities that are performed at a higher intensity, such as bicycling, jumping rope, running, shoveling snow, or climbing stairs for a shorter amount of time (fifteen minutes or so) to get similar results. However, it is not necessary to do high-intensity exercises to achieve health benefits, particularly those associated with improvements in cholesterol levels. Moderate-intensity exercise can improve heart health. The most important thing is to get moving!

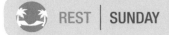

"Don't pray when it rains if you don't pray when the sun shines."

—Satchel Paige

Recite a Prayer or Make Up Your Own

Harold Koenig, MD, associate professor of psychiatry and medicine at Duke University School of Medicine in Durham, North Carolina, has observed that religious people tend to have healthier lives. But prayer does not solely belong to those who consider themselves "religious" or someone who belongs to a church or participates in organized religion. Prayer can be a quiet meditation in which you ask for guidance, or strength, or faith—from a divinity, from the universe, or from within. Even if you are not religious, prayer can center you when things are not going right in your life, give solace and lift you when you feel down, and remind you that you aren't alone. Praying can help you move forward when you feel stuck or provide hope when you need healing. Recite a prayer that gives you comfort. Or, if you prefer you can make up your own prayer. A simple "thank you" is a powerful prayer of gratitude. "I need your help" or "Please guide me" are also excellent points of departure into prayer. Pray and then be still like an empty vessel waiting to be filled. Gratefully receive whatever inspiration, answers, relief, peace, joy, and bliss may come.

"Our research shows that people may have a better outcome losing weight if they increase their intake of lean protein."

—Osama Hamdy, MD, PhD

Eat More Lean Protein

Proteins, which are made up of amino acids, work within the body as primary building blocks for all tissues and cells, including your muscles. Their secondary function is to provide energy after your carbohydrate resources have been depleted—thereby boosting your metabolism! One gram of protein equals 4 calories and it can be found in meat, fish, eggs, dairy, and legumes (beans and peas). While legumes are low in fat and high in fiber, animal sources of protein can be higher in unwanted fats yet also provide necessary amino acids, so you may want to alternate the two for maximum benefit.

Your body has to work twice as hard to digest protein as carbohydrates or fats, which means your metabolism has to work harder, too. Also, a study published in the *American Journal of Clinical Nutrition* found that when people ate more protein and cut down on fat, they reduced their calorie intake by 441 calories a day. In fact, experts think that eating protein actually enhances the effect of leptin, a hormone that helps the body feel full. When you choose protein, reach for the healthier choices, such as fish, skinless chicken, lean pork, tofu, nuts, beans, eggs, and low-fat dairy products, with the occasional lean red meat.

WEEK SEVEN

"Muscular strength is essential for a high level of performance in many sports and activities. There are many other health factors that come along with strength training as well. Strong muscles help keep joints strong, making them less susceptible to sprains, strains, and other injuries."

—Tina Angelotti, developer of Krav Maga fitness program

Determine Your One-Repetition Maximum

The formal definition of muscular strength is the ability of a muscle or group of muscles to generate maximal force. The test for determining your maximum strength is referred to as the one-repetition maximum, or the 1-RM. To determine your 1-RM, select a weight that you know you can lift or press at least once. After a proper warm-up, perform a few repetitions. If you are successful, add some more weight and try again. Repeat this until you are unable to move the weight more than one repetition. The weight you are able to do only one repetition with is considered your 1-RM and is a measurement of your muscular strength. Record this number in a journal, and upon the completion of thirty days of training repeat this test and see how much your strength has improved.

DEVELOPING MAXIMUM STRENGTH

In general, exercises with so much resistance that you are unable to exceed a minimum of twelve repetitions are the kinds of exercises that build muscular strength. Power lifters, at one extreme, often work with weights that are heavy enough to limit their sets to four or fewer reps, and they often perform six to ten sets. This type of training effectively develops the greatest potential for maximum strength.

"I read Freud's Introductory Lectures in Psychoanalysis *in basically one sitting. I decided to enroll in medical school. It was almost like a conversion experience."*

—Stanislav Grof

Attend Lectures

Lectures offer incredible opportunities to learn, to acquire new interests, stay current, and improve your conversational skills. Pick topics that you know nothing about—like neuroscience, archeology, quantum physics, ancient history, hieroglyphics, etc.—and charge up your brain cells by straining to understand. The more complex the subject matter, the more it generates new thoughts and gets your brainwaves sparking. Many universities, libraries, and organizations offer free lectures and local newspapers or news channel websites are great resources for finding them. When you find something that sounds intriguing, call a few friends and invite them to come along. That way you can have a stimulating conversation afterward. Or, if you go alone, strike up conversations and make new friends.

Some subjects we found recently:

- "Incognito: The Secret Life of the Brain"
- "Exceptional Animals: Sponges as Oracles of the History of Life"
- "Consciousness, Creativity, and the Brain, presented by filmmaker David Lynch"

"As you age, you lose range of motion, and your muscles lose flexibility. Failing to stretch is inviting disaster."

—Lucia Colbert, participant in over 100 triathlons

Know the Dos and Don'ts of Stretching

You can do more harm than good if you do your stretching the wrong way. Here are stretch principles that will be of benefit to you as you intensify your endurance-building workouts.

Do:

- Warm up before stretching. This cannot be overemphasized.
- Hold most stretches for at least twenty seconds.
- Stretch daily. If necessary, take ten minutes off one of your workouts to make time for stretching. It's that important.
- Be careful about stretching outside in very cold weather. For example, when there's snow on the ground, take extra time to warm up before you try to stretch.
- Take a deep breath before you begin the stretch.
- Exhale as you stretch the muscle. This practice allows the spine to increase flexion, which enhances the effectiveness of the stretch.
- Focus on problem areas and stretch the tighter side more if there is an imbalance.

Don't:

- Bounce when stretching. You should maintain a constant tension on the muscle. Bouncing can cause injury.
- Push to keep stretching when it hurts to do so. At most, the tension in the muscle should be mild discomfort. It should never hurt.
- Stretch injured muscles.

- Stretch cold muscles. Always warm up before stretching. This can be done with as little as a ten-minute walk or five-minute jog. You risk injury when you try to stretch cold muscles.
- Forget to stretch opposing muscle groups. Stretching one side but not the other can lead to imbalances that cause injuries.
- Forget to stretch the upper body as well as the legs.

"Dance is bigger than the physical body. When you extend your arm, it doesn't stop at the end of your fingers, because you're dancing bigger than that; you're dancing spirit."

—Judith Jamison

Take a Dance Class

Dance is a fabulous way to increase flexibility. Most dance classes focus on stretching and increasing flexibility because dancing itself requires you to move your body in new and unusual ways—unless you're already a ballet dancer or professional dancer. Luckily, many dance studios and gyms offer dance classes for beginner adults, and the classes are not competitive in nature. Everyone generally comes to have fun, learn something new, and limber up his or her body.

No matter what form of dance you take (ballet, jazz, ballroom, hip hop, modern, or other), the instructor should lead you in stretching exercises that target all the main muscle groups in your body. As we've already emphasized in Week Three, stretching is one of the most important things you can do to increase your overall flexibility, and repeat stretching will lead to greater flexibility over time.

Now get out there and have some fun!

"A bookstore is one of the only pieces of evidence we have that people are still thinking."

—Jerry Seinfeld

Spend the Afternoon at a Bookstore or Coffee Shop

Book lovers adore bookstores. They also enjoy a cup of good coffee or tea while they read. It's no accident that while many book shops have added refreshment areas where you can purchase a cup of your favorite coffee or tea, coffee houses also sell newspapers and, in some cases, books that the shop is promoting. So, if books are your thing, head off for a delightful afternoon of reading and sipping at a local bookstore. Get to know others who share your passion for literature. It's a good thing to widen your circle of friends. Happiness is doing what you love with others who love doing the things you do.

WHILE YOU'RE THERE, READ THE CLASSICS

Reading is great for brain health, particularly if you focus on works that challenge you. The latest potboiler may be a fun read, but it's probably as mentally challenging as a Dick and Jane primer. You can give your brain a workout by reading a literary classic you've always meant to tackle or by reading a nonfiction book on a topic you're interested in but know nothing about. Read carefully, with memory and recall in mind. To help you assimilate this new information, discuss it with friends.

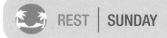
> *"A man with one watch knows what time it is; a man*
> *with two watches is never quite sure."*
>
> —Lee Segall

Simplify Your Life

To make your home a less stressful, more tranquil place, one of the easiest things you can do is to simplify. Spend some time in each room of your home and list all the things you do in each room. What are the functions of the room? What is impeding that function? And what would make each room simpler, its functions simpler?

Simplify your cleaning chores by creating a system for getting everything done a little bit each day. Simplify your shopping by buying in bulk and by planning your menu a week in advance. You can simplify the way your home works and consequently reduce your stress while in your home in many ways. Many excellent books, magazines, and websites are devoted to simple living. See the resource list at the end of this book for further reading. Here are some more simplicity tips for your home:

- Wear your clothes a little longer (unless they get stained) to cut down on laundry.
- Choose a wardrobe in which everything matches.
- Change your bedding less often. Who's going to notice?
- Get rid of or pack away household items that complicate your life without giving you very much back—ornate items that require constant dusting, house plants that require constant watering, dishes you can't put in the dishwasher, clothes you have to have dry-cleaned.
- Hire a student or a neighboring teenager to mow the lawn, rake the leaves, run errands, or baby-sit. Consider hiring a housecleaning service.

There are always more ways to simplify. Keep looking for them.

"Don't dig your grave with your own knife and fork."

—English Proverb

Choose Whole Grains Over Refined Grains

Foods made from grains should be the base of a nutritious diet. Grains include bread, rice, pasta, and oats. Whole-grain foods, especially unprocessed whole grains, supply vitamin E and B vitamins such as folic acid, as well as minerals like magnesium, iron, and zinc. Whole grains (like whole wheat) are rich in fiber and higher in other important nutrients. In fact, eating plenty of whole-grain breads, bran cereals, and other whole-grain foods can easily provide half of your fiber needs for an entire day.

Refined grains include white bread and white rice. Whole grain is the entire edible part of any grain, including wheat, corn, oats, and rice. Refined grains go through a milling process in which parts of the grain are removed. In refined grains, many of the essential nutrients are lost in processing. Some nutrients are added back, or the product is enriched, but this usually does not include all of the nutrients that were lost.

The aim should be to consume at least six servings of grain products per day. When choosing grains, words such as whole grain, whole wheat, rye, bulgur, brown rice, oatmeal, whole oats, pearl barley, and whole-grain corn should be one of the first words in the ingredient list on a food label. The best whole-grain or whole-wheat products are made from 100 percent whole-wheat flour. Choose grains that are rich in fiber, low in saturated fat, and low in sodium.

WEEK EIGHT

"It's always challenging to start something new. Be sure to give yourself plenty of credit. You deserve it. And, every weight that you lift, even if it's only 5 pounds to start with, is important. It is leading you on the road towards a healthier, stronger, and more active lifestyle."

—Shirley S. Archer, fitness professional, Stanford University School of Medicine

Select the Right Weight Load

The weight load that you choose for weight lifting determines the number of reps that you can do. The best way to find a proper weight level for you is initially through trial and error. Always start out on the conservative side with a weight you think might be light for you.

If you can lift this weight easily for 15 reps, then it's too light. If you lifted between 16 to 17 reps, go ahead and add 5 pounds. If you lifted between 18 and 19 reps, try adding 10 pounds. If you easily lifted more than 20 reps, see how you do with an additional 15 pounds.

If you can successfully complete 12 to 15 reps in your first attempt, then this is your training load. You can note this on your exercise log. As you become more experienced, you will remember how much weight you lift on each of the exercises. When you're starting out, however, it can feel much more like information overload. Write it down. You will save plenty of time on your next workouts.

What if, in spite of your best efforts to select a weight on the light side, you discover that you can not even lift 12 reps? This weight level is too heavy. Save it for another day when you are stronger. If you could only lift between 10 to 11 reps, subtract 5 pounds. If you completed between 8 and 9 reps, go ahead and lower the weight by 10 pounds. If you really overestimated your own strength and could not even lift 7 reps, don't worry. You will become stronger if you stick with your program. We guarantee it. In the meantime, drop down at least 15 pounds and be proud that you are starting out with a program—and keep up the great work!

"What soap is to the body, laughter is to the soul."

—Yiddish Proverb

Watch a Funny Movie

Laugh! It really is the best medicine—for both our minds and our bodies. For one thing, a good sense of humor provides needed stress relief. When we laugh at our problems rather than fret over them, they become less serious and thus easier to solve. Humor also improves cognitive function by keeping the mind active and encouraging creative thinking—a vital defense against age—and provides an important emotional catharsis during periods of emotional tension. Researchers at Loma Linda University School of Medicine's Department of Clinical Immunology conducted numerous studies proving that laughter helps lower serum cortisol levels, increases the amount of activated T lymphocytes, increases the number and activity of natural killer cells, and increases the number of T cells that have helper/suppressor receptors. In other words, laughter helps stimulate the immune system and counters the immunosuppressive effects of stress. Laughter also benefits the heart, improves oxygen flow to the brain, and works the muscles in the head, neck, chest, and pelvis—in much the same way as the stress reduction exercises of yoga. This helps keep muscles loose and limber and enables them to rest more easily. So rent a funny movie, go to a comedy club, or watch a comedy show and laugh!

"I go running when I have to. When the ice cream truck is doing sixty."

—Wendy Liebman

Create a Training Log

Another item that will improve your running experience is a training log. Use a notebook, calendar, or running log to record the following information at a minimum: miles run, total time run, and shoe model worn. Some runners record everything from the weather conditions to the route they have run to the total shoe mileage.

Keeping a log is important because it provides a history of your running, which is crucial for finding the possible cause of a running injury. Additionally, reviewing a running log helps to determine the training method that has been most effective in turning out your best performances. Finally, keeping a log is highly motivating, for few runners like to leave too many blank entries. However, do not become compulsive about your running just to fill in the blanks or reach a specific weekly mileage total come what may.

A training log may not seem like an essential item in your quest for fitness, but it is. It's a place to set goals, track achievements, and note ups or downs. You'll be thrilled to look back at the mileage you've run, and in turn you'll be more motivated to stick to your plan.

There are a variety of websites that provide training logs and show you how to record everything pertaining to your training program, from actual miles run to cumulative shoe mileage. Best of all, most of these sites are free.

"All those years of skating and dancing have carried over.
I can't design anything without thinking of how a woman's
body will look and move when she's wearing it."

—Vera Wang

Take an Aerobics Dance Class

Just as happened in the 1980s, aerobics classes with dance influences are all the rage. Zumba, for instance, has become one of the hottest crazes in group fitness classes. A lively workout, it combines Latin dance-inspired movements with cardiovascular activity. Zumba is an especially good class to take for improving flexibility, but any form of dance aerobics would be beneficial.

Like all other dance and cardio classes, Zumba involves an extensive warm-up and cool-down section that begins with plenty of stretching. Because it's a class for all levels, you can ease into the movements and dance at your own pace. The combination of lunges, squats, hip swirls, and shoulder rolls, among other movements, will increase your flexibility dramatically, often without you feeling the type of repetitive drudgery that less exciting workouts often bring.

While easing in is highly recommended, if you want to see drastic improvement in your overall flexibility, you have to be willing to push yourself a little past your comfort zone when you stretch—and when you're out there on the floor. Rest assured that with time, your body will feel more and more limber. Classes are widely available and you usually don't have to join a gym to participate in classes.

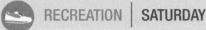

> *"The sovereign invigorator of the body is exercise,*
> *and of all the exercises walking is the best."*
>
> —Thomas Jefferson

Take 10,000 Steps a Day

Many people are now trying to ensure they take at least 10,000 steps per day, which has been shown to be a marker of good health. If you walk about 3.5 miles per hour, then you probably take somewhere between 5,000 and 7,000 steps in one hour, depending on your height (and, therefore, your stride length). You can walk that number of steps during a one-hour show on TV just by marching in front of your TV. You'll burn about 150 to 250 calories during that hour. That may not sound like a lot, but if you're just watching TV without moving, you'll only burn about 40 to 60 calories, and not get any boost to your metabolism during that time. Do that for one hour a day for a year, and you'll burn off about 9 pounds!

Of course, you can also buy a step counter, or pedometer, which you can hook onto your pants (at the waistband) or your shoes. These little doodads, which have become so popular that McDonald's was giving them away for a while, are supposed to be an easy way to help you make sure you're getting your 10,000 steps in. The problem is that these machines are often inaccurate, so they either overcount or undercount your steps. Nevertheless, they aren't expensive and they do work for some people, so you might try one out. Take 100 steps (count), and then see how close the piece of equipment is. If it's pretty close (maybe 95 to 105 steps) then use it. If not, try to make estimates yourself.

"I like nonsense, it wakes up the brain cells. Fantasy is a necessary ingredient in living, it's a way of looking at life through the wrong end of a telescope. Which is what I do, and that enables you to laugh at life's realities."

—Theodore Geisel

Take a Mental Vacation

For instant relaxation, imagery can work for you. Imagery is simple and fun. Feeling stressed? Feeling anxious? Feeling hopeless? Go on vacation. No, don't leave your desk and head to the airport. Stay at your desk, close your eyes, relax, breathe, and use your imagination to visualize the place you would most like to be.

You remember your imagination, don't you? It was that thing that, as a child, allowed you to fly like a bird, stomp like an elephant, bark like a dog, save the world from disaster, go on safari, jump from an airplane with your parachute, and visit a land made entirely out of candy, all in one day. Remember that? Wasn't that fun?

Your imagination is still in your head, even if it's grown a little rusty from disuse. Time to take it out, brush it off, and use it in the service of stress management! You might not decide to imagine that you are a superhero (then again, you might, and why not?), but why not imagine wandering down a secluded beach at sunset, the balmy tropical winds rippling the turquoise sea? Maybe you would prefer cuddling in front of the fire with a special someone (even if you haven't met him or her yet) in a cozy cabin in the woods? Maybe images of the Far East, the rain forest, or hiking a glacier in Alaska invoke a sense of peace in you. Maybe you're partial to the desert . . . or a really fancy dessert!

Let yourself daydream a little. Consider it personal time. Time to recharge. It's fun, and it's perfectly legal. It's also an excellent way to manage the stress that comes your way. After all, that's what vacations are for!

"The goal is to have as little trans fat in your diet as possible."

—Cindy Moore, MS, RD, director of nutrition therapy,
Cleveland Clinic Foundation

Severely Limit Foods Containing Artificial Trans Fat

Artificial trans fat is produced when liquid vegetable oil is treated with heat, chemicals, and hydrogen to transform it into a product that is semisolid at room temperature. Food producers began using it because it's inexpensive, performs beautifully in both baked and deep-fried applications, keeps food fresher longer, and provides a nice "mouthfeel" to many products—but artificial trans fats are also one of the few food ingredients that is truly bad for you.

Basically, your body doesn't recognize these trans fats as an artificial substance, so doesn't discard it in the digestion process. Instead, it is used in chemical reactions as though it was a normal fatty acid. In your cell membranes, in the lining of arteries and veins, and in your liver, brain, and kidneys, trans fat is fully incorporated, changing the functions and properties of your cells and of the enzymes that fuel your body. Sometimes knowing how something affects your body inspires you to eat healthier. Trans fat has been proven to affect our bodies negatively in the following ways:

- Increases LDL cholesterol levels
- Decreases HDL cholesterol levels
- Damages cell membranes, decreasing nutrient absorption
- Reduces flexibility of capillaries and arteries
- Increases the level of insulin in the bloodstream
- Contributes to weight gain, especially around the midsection
- Causes inflammation in cell walls and artery walls
- Increases the risk of cancer through free radicals

Foods high in trans fats include: margarine, fast food, baked goods, chips, crackers, cookies, and candy.

"Great changes may not happen right away, but with effort even the difficult may become easy."

—Bill Blackman

Add Weight Training to Build Greater Strength

Whether you are young or old, heavy or lean, a long-distance runner or a sprinter, you will benefit from weight training, also known as strength training. The increase in lean muscle mass that results from strength training is key to overall strength and to your body's ability to burn calories. This is because muscle cells require more energy (and also burn more calories) than fat cells. Overall fitness requires more than just cardiovascular fitness. A balance of endurance, strength, and flexibility must be achieved. The most often recognized components of fitness include:

- Muscular fitness, strength, and endurance
- Flexibility
- Cardiovascular endurance
- Balanced nutrition
- Body composition

The last item, body composition, acts as a guide to how your body is doing overall, but it is not a pure component of fitness. Although running is one of the best cardiovascular activities, other than strengthening a few specific muscles and rapidly burning a lot of calories, it does not fulfill many of the other criteria of overall fitness, which is why weight training is essential to your overall health.

"Thought is cause, experience is effect. If you don't like the effects in your life, you have to change the nature of your thinking."

—Marianne Williamson

Think Positively

According to Daniel G. Amen, MD, author of *Making a Good Brain Great*, every thought releases brain chemicals. Positive, happy, hopeful, optimistic, joyful thoughts produce yummy chemicals that create a sense of well-being and help your brain function at peak capacity; unhappy, miserable, negative, dark thoughts have the opposite effect, effectively slowing down your brain and even creating depression. If you tend to focus on what can go wrong, or what is wrong, or how unhappy you are, or how someone hurt you, these negative thoughts can dim your brain's capacity to function. It saps the brain of its positive forcefulness. Dr. Amen suggests writing out negative thoughts to dispel their power over your brain.

A HAPPY BRAIN IS AN ENERGETIC BRAIN

Thinking patterns have been shown to affect brain activity and negative thinking has been shown to affect the brain in negative ways. Negative thinking slows down brain coordination, making it difficult to process thoughts and find solutions. Feeling frightened, which often happens when focused on negative outcomes, has been shown to decrease activity in the cerebellum, which slows the brain's ability to process new information, and the left temporal lobe, which affects mood, memory, and impulse control.

"People who shop in health food stores never look healthy."

—Amy Sedaris

Make Sure Your Diet Is Supporting Your Endurance Training

Nutrition is one of the most important considerations you face when intensifying your workouts to build endurance. Eating right is a major contributor to your overall comfort level and enhanced performance. Building endurance requires rigorous activities that stress muscles and longer and more intense workouts that can frequently lead to injury, if you don't take precautions. Preventive medicine, for example, holds that if you take steps to avoid injury, it is less likely to occur. Another preventive measure is to provide for your body from the inside out: Feed your body what it needs to work to capacity, and it will be better able to perform. To that end, nutritional therapy can help. This includes:

- A regular source of high-quality protein as part of your meals.
- Vitamin C to support healing, reduce swelling, repair tissue, and keep ligaments and tendons strong.
- Calcium and magnesium as essential for bone and muscle health.
- Bromelain to help reduce swelling, especially when taken with turmeric.
- Zinc as important for bone health and tissue repair.
- Omega-3 fatty acids, such as flax and fish oils, as natural anti-inflammatories.

"Forget your opponents; always play against par."

—Sam Snead

Play Golf

Most people (who don't play golf) think that golf doesn't require a lot of athletic prowess or offer a lot of exercise. It does appear to be a low-level physical activity, especially if you use a golf cart. However, golf actually requires a fairly high level of physical fitness—especially flexibility. When playing golf, every single muscle has to work properly and work together to execute the perfect golf swing. Although it may not look like you need to be very flexible to swing a golf club, the truth is that you need a solid combination of strength and balance to power a golf ball long distances, with maximum accuracy. Even putting requires good elasticity in your muscles to twist and turn your body correctly. From your hands and wrists that help grip the golf club, to your hips that help create the acceleration of the golf club, to your feet that help swing through the golf ball, flexibility is one of the most underrated aspects of the game of golf.

Outside of just feeling better on the golf course, flexibility has some real benefits to it. For one, you can improve muscle elasticity and blood circulation throughout your body. You can also prevent injuries to your arms, shoulders, wrists, hips, back, and legs. If you want to improve at golf, work on your flexibility by taking it to the club often.

"No pleasure endures unseasoned by variety."

—Syrus (Publilius Syrus)

Add Variety to Your Daily Activities

When it comes to exercise, it's always good to have a variety of options. Doing so means that you'll be working different muscles and alternating intensity. When it comes to recreational exercise, variety keeps it interesting—and works different sets of muscles and builds different sets of skills. Maybe you want to take a country line or ballroom dancing class one night a week, then join a mountain-biking, birdwatching, hiking, or dog-walking club that gets you out of the house a few nights a week. You could add long walks or bicycle rides or even gardening another evening, and hiking on Sundays. Just as it's important that you enjoy your exercise regimen, because it reduces the chances that you'll get bored and quit, it's also important to have a wide variety of nourishing, fun activities that keep you energized, enthusiastic, and happy.

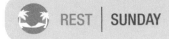

"As we free our breath (through diaphragmatic breathing)
we relax our emotions and let go our body tensions."

—Gay Hendricks

Learn to Take Complete Breaths

Most of us rely on shallow breaths (ones that don't progress beyond the lungs), when what our bodies need for rejuvenation and energy is deep breathing. Here's how to deepen your breaths: Lie down with bent knees, and begin breathing through your nostrils and observing your breath. Become aware of the natural length of your inhalation and exhalation, and the pauses in between. Remain relaxed, without changing or forcing the breath. Let the breath flow smoothly and evenly. Relax your facial muscles and jaw.

Now place your hands on your lower abdomen, allowing them to rest there lightly. As you breathe in, feel your hands fill with your breath as your belly gently expands. Notice how your belly contracts, moving away from your hands and receding into your body upon exhalation. Spend ten to twelve breaths observing the movement of the breath in your belly.

Next, lightly place your palms on your lower, front, floating ribs. Let your wrists relax down to your body. Again, let the breath come into your hands upon inhalation and feel your ribs contracting on exhalation. Do this for another ten to twelve breaths.

Lastly, place your hands on your collarbones and observe the breath filling the area under your hands on the inhalation. Notice how your top chest recedes with the exhalation. Practice this for ten to twelve breaths.

Then allow your arms to come back to your sides, palms facing up. Continue to watch your breath, feeling the three-part breathing pattern. You may find that the breath comes in more easily to one area than it does to another. For example, many people find it difficult, initially, to fill the top chest on inhalation. Over time and with practice, you will be able to breathe more fully and deeply, filling your entire body with the breath.

"A mind of the caliber of mine cannot derive its nutriment from cows."

—George Bernard Shaw

Eat More Fish

Fish and shellfish are excellent sources of protein that are also low in fat. One serving (3 ounces) of most fish and shellfish provides about 20 grams of protein, which is approximately one third of the recommended daily amount for the average adult. In addition, fish contain all of the essential amino acid our bodies need to function and have other important minerals like iron, zinc, and, in those fish with edible bones, calcium.

As you may know, fish are also rich in omega-3 fatty acids, which promote the development of healthy membranes that make it easier for your body to use stored fat and sugar for energy. Even better, those who dine often on fish may have more leptin in their system, a hormone linked with high metabolism, appetite control, and weight loss.

The American Heart Association recommends that you eat fish rich in omega-3 fatty acids (mackerel, lake trout, herring, sardines, albacore tuna, and salmon) at least twice a week in order to reap all of its benefits.

WEEK TEN

CATCH SOME TUNA . . . IN MODERATION

It's not a coincidence that 90 percent of all bodybuilders and fitness competitors in the world will tell you they make a habit of feasting on tuna. They know it's an excellent source of protein that offers very few calories and almost no fat. These people need to be lean to compete, and tuna is often their answer. Caution: Eat tuna in moderation (once or twice a week) because it can be high in mercury. Alternate it with other fish, such as salmon.

"If your [weight-lifting] goal is basic conditioning and you are training for the first time, it's generally recommended that you start out with a lower intensity."

—Shirley S. Archer, fitness professional, Stanford University School of Medicine

Start Out with One-Set Training

When you first begin a weight-training program, your body is working hard. You are conditioning your joints so that they can become accustomed to the challenge of extra weight. You are developing an important network of neuromuscular pathways from your brain, through your spinal column, and into your muscles. It takes time to build this network!

Think of your body as an organic electronic circuit board. All of the wiring needs to be laid into place. Each time you perform an exercise movement, you are firing up the circuit board. The organic circuit board gets stronger with use over time. Respect the process. Give your body time to adjust and you will reap rewards.

Start out lifting weights that make you feel tired when you reach between the eighth to twelfth repetition. Work up to twelve repetitions. Consider one set sufficient to start. After you have worked out comfortably for a few weeks at twelve repetitions per set, go ahead and add a second set. Once you've mastered 12 to 15 reps to fatigue, you can then progress to two sets at that level. After you've mastered two sets at the 12- to 15-rep level, then you can progress to one set at a heavier weight level (no more than 5 percent) in the 8- to 12-rep range. If that's too much, then increase the weight level but continue to work in the 12- to 15-rep range. In this way, you can gradually and progressively build strength. Remember, always increase reps first, and then add an additional set.

"I can get a better grasp of what is going on in the world from one good Washington dinner party than from all the background information NBC piles on my desk."

—Barbara Walters

Host Dinner Parties

Dinner parties offer great opportunities to socialize and to discuss a wide range of topics in depth. Invite friends and acquaintances from all walks of life and play your part as host or hostess by encouraging stimulating conversation. Bone up on your guests' professions and be ready to introduce controversial or exciting topics that will engage your mind—and those of your guests. Your guests and your brain will thank you for it.

Here are a few ideas for thematic dinner parties:

- Murder Mystery Dinner Parties. These have become very popular because they're such fun—and they involve everyone in the game. You'll find lots of resources online for plotting your party—and the imaginary murder.
- Wine Tasting Dinner. You can have fun planning the menu and selecting the wine pairings. Your memory will get a workout when you call upon your research to offer up tidbits about each wine to your friends. Look for obscure, interesting facts about each wine or winery to share and do your best to commit them to memory.
- Philosopher's Night Out. Invite friends to pick their favorite philosopher (dead or living, traditional or wacky) and have each speak for five minutes on their selection and why they particularly admire his or her ideas. This will spark lots of conversation. For extra fun, have each guest keep his choice a secret to see if anyone can guess the identity.
- Trivia Night. Everyone loves obscure facts. Play the game before settling in for dinner and everyone's tongues will still be wagging when dessert is served.

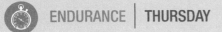

"When I first started running, I was so embarrassed I'd walk when cars passed me. I'd pretend I was looking at flowers."

—Joan Benoit Samuelson, Olympic medalist

Follow the 10 Percent Rule

It's hard not to feel like you can strap on your running shoes and do 5 miles easily. Although it's admirable to want to seize the day, remember, slow and steady wins the race. You'll be running an easy 5 miles soon enough if you train smart.

In building your mileage base, remember the 10 percent rule: Do not increase either your weekly mileage and/or your long-run mileage by more than 10 percent a week. Doing so greatly increases the chance of incurring an injury, thereby delaying or stopping your training altogether. This is one of the biggest mistakes runners make. Don't do it!

Without a doubt, runners—particularly those running to build endurance—should include supplemental activities such as weight training and cross-training as part of their total fitness program. In particular, incorporating weight training, stretching, and carefully selected cross-training activities in your fitness regimen both reduces the risk of injury and facilitates total-body conditioning.

'JUST SAY NO' TO MARATHONS

You shouldn't even think of training for a marathon (26.2 miles) until meeting certain conditions. Specifically, you should have been running consistently four to five days per week, 25 miles per week, for at least a year (without any major injuries).

"The calming, relaxing feeling Tai Chi creates is great stress relief. It's really about restoring all your body's systems to an optimal level of performance."

—Michael Clark, Tai Chi and Qigong teacher

Explore Tai Chi

Tai Chi and its precursor, Qigong, are ancient Chinese Taoist martial arts forms that have evolved to fit the twenty-first century. Rarely used today as a method of defense, Tai Chi consists of a series of slow, graceful movements in concert with the breath designed to free internal energy and keep it flowing through the body, uniting body and mind, promoting good health and relaxation. Tai Chi is sometimes called a moving meditation.

The individual Tai Chi movements are called forms, and each form often recalls an animal or something in nature, such as a tree or reed. Some form names include "Grasp the bird's tail" and "Wave hands like clouds." These names are evocative of the movement, which incorporate all the limbs and the breath.

Research on Tai Chi has found it to be helpful for mood disorders, such as anxiety and depression, as well as physical ailments, such as arthritis and hypertension. Because you perform Tai Chi while standing and use your whole body, it can build muscular strength and slightly increase cardiovascular function. More than anything, though, Tai Chi is great for balance training, flexibility, and relaxation. Because Tai Chi has grown in popularity, you may be able to locate classes near to your home or place of business online.

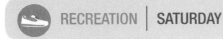

"A friend knows the song in my heart and sings it to me when my memory fails."

—Donna Roberts

Sing Your Heart Out

Singing has been connected to intelligence, creativity, emotion, and memory, according to Daniel G. Amen, author of *Making a Good Brain Great*. It has been proven that singing information or attaching a melody or jingle to it helps you retain the information. "Singing stimulates temporal lobe function, an area of the brain heavily involved in memory," Dr. Amen reported. If you can't sing, try humming, which Dr. Amen said also provides a positive difference in mood and memory. "As the sound activates your brain, you will feel more alive and your brain will feel more tuned in to the moment."

WHEN YOU CAN'T SING, LISTEN TO MUSIC

Researchers have found that the same pleasure centers of the brain that are positively stimulated by food and sex are also affected by music. Any music that sends chills up your spine has a direct effect upon your mood. When we use music that is particularly stimulating to us in a positive way, we can elevate our mood, and feel more content, relaxed, energized, or turned on.

"The body never lies."

—Martha Graham

Make Self-Care a Priority

One of the biggest contributors to feelings of stress is the sense that life is out of control. To avoid this, make time for yourself, just like taking time to exercise or eat healthy. You deserve time for your own self-care. For one thing, it supports your health, which in turn helps you to better support those you care about. Take a moment to identify things that you enjoy, that bring you pleasure, and that are fun and restorative. Make it a point to incorporate these activities into your schedule.

It is never easy to change a habit. Unless stress is managed and the reasons for maintaining the behavioral change are foremost in your mind, old habits prevail. A calm, clear, and focused mind and a healthy, realistic attitude are important for achieving any goal. This holds equally true for the incorporation of healthy lifestyle habits.

WHY BEING ABLE TO RELAX IS VITAL TO YOUR HEALTH

Research suggests that relaxation techniques can be used to counteract the stress response, with significant health benefits. Regular relaxation can reduce blood cortisol levels, blood pressure, cholesterol, and blood glucose. Clinical trials show that relaxation can reduce headaches, pain, anxiety, and menopausal symptoms. At the same time, it can enhance healing, immune cell response, concentration, and feelings of well-being. It has even been shown to improve fertility rates in infertile women.

"A nickel's worth of goulash beats a five-dollar can of vitamins."

—Martin H. Fischer

Eat Nutrient-Rich Vegetables

Some foods are better for you than others. Fruits and vegetables, for example, are an important part of any health regimen because they are loaded with essential nutrients in their most natural and useful form—and the more fruits and vegetables you eat the more satiated you will feel and you will be able to avoid high-calorie foods and fat.

In fact, many vegetables will satisfy—or nearly satisfy—your daily requirements for several vitamins. From dark leafy greens rich in calcium, iron, and magnesium to the cruciferous vegetables like bok choy, broccoli, cabbage, turnips, and water cress that have cancer-preventing antioxidants to nutrient-rich vegetables like carrots, potatoes, yams, and tomatoes, vegetables are always a good thing to snack on and include with each meal.

The majority of Americans don't consume nearly enough fruits and vegetables. Government health officials suggest a minimum of five servings of fruit and vegetables daily—twice the amount suggested for meat and dairy.

WEEK ELEVEN

BUY LOCAL ORGANIC VEGETABLES

If you buy organic produce, you'll also get more nutritional bang from your buck if you buy produce that was grown locally or regionally. Experts agree that fruits, vegetables, and greens provide peak nutrition when they are ripe. Unfortunately, more than 60 percent of the commercial produce in the United States is picked before it's ripe, which means the produce you buy at traditional grocery stores doesn't have its full nutritional component.

"Many advanced bodybuilders divide their body parts into two groups and exercise them alternately on consecutive days. This is known as working a 'split routine.'"

—Shirley S. Archer, fitness professional, Stanford University School of Medicine

Schedule Two Days a Week for Weight-Lifting Workouts

The American College of Sports Medicine (ACSM) recommends that you train a minimum of two times a week. Why at least twice a week? You need to stimulate your muscles regularly to gain improvements. Why not more frequently? You can train more often, but research shows that increasing the frequency of training results in a minimal amount of additional improvement relative to the additional time investment.

In other words, the most bang for your buck comes from those first two days a week. More days of exercise will give you more bang, just not as big a bang. To quantify this difference, according to research studies, training two days a week may produce only 75 percent of the gains that a three-day-a-week program would. So it's really up to you and what you want. The bottom line is that a minimum amount of strength training will result in significant health and fitness improvements.

WHY YOU NEED TO LIMIT WORKOUTS

As with many things in life, when it comes to weight training, more is not necessarily better. Muscles need at least forty-eight hours in between training sessions to recover and repair. If you're training your entire body daily, your muscles will not have time to build new tissue.

"I am the one who got myself fat, who did all the eating.
So I had to take full responsibility for it."

—Kirstie Alley

Keep Your Brain Supple by Eating a Low-Fat Diet

Improperly stored oils and fats will go rancid, and that's just what happens in your body when you eat a high-fat diet. Since the brain and nervous system are very high in fat, some researchers speculate that rancid fat may be damaging the brain by causing free radicals (unstable molecules that potentially cause cell damage). Scientists have discovered that eating a diet in which 40 percent of the calories come from fat raises the risk of Alzheimer's in someone who has the ApoE4 gene an incredible twenty-nine times. Younger people aged twenty to thirty-nine with the ApoE4 gene are twenty-three times more likely to develop Alzheimer's in later years than are healthy eaters.

Fat intake should not exceed 15 to 20 percent of your total calories, but the quality of the fat is even more important. Essentially, omega-3 fats are excellent; trans fats are damaging.

CUT WAY BACK ON THE BAD FATS

American diets tend to be overabundant in saturated, hydrogenated, and partially hydrogenated trans fats. Saturated fats tend to raise cholesterol levels and thus endanger your heart and your brain. Saturated fats are usually solid at room temperature and can be found in well-marbled meat, butter, whole milk cheese, ice cream, egg yolks, and fatty cuts of beef, pork, and lamb. Trans fats may be even more harmful than saturated and hydrogenated fats. They disrupt the production of energy in the mitochondria (the energy factories) of brain cells. When it comes to trans fats, just say no.

"I thought about how many preconceived prejudices would crumble when I trotted right along for 26 miles."

—Roberta "Bobbi" Gibb, first woman to run the Boston Marathon (1966)

Buy Yourself a Running Watch

You will come to depend on your running watch the way you depend on your wristwatch when you think you might be late for work. Your running watch will let you know how you're doing at all times.

The watch you use doesn't have to be expensive (though it can be). Before purchasing a watch for running, decide what functions you think you'll really use. Most include a stopwatch, an alarm, lap settings (also called split timing), a glow light for seeing your time at night, and a regular watch. Make sure the model you choose isn't too complicated or intimidating. The stopwatch will be the part you use most, so make sure it's easy to start, stop, and reset, and is also waterproof.

But why simply monitor your overall time and distance when you can learn so much more about your performance during a run? There are a variety of models that enable you to continuously monitor your speed, distance, pace, calories burned, and heart rate throughout the various phases of your workout. You can even make your workouts more challenging with a virtual partner feature, enabling you to train alongside a digital competitor with programmable specified time, distance, and pace goals. Some devices feature the capability of downloading information to a computer so you can both store the data and keep an online running log (see Week Eight).

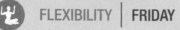

"Gymnastics uses every single part of your body,
every little tiny muscle that you never even knew."

—Shannon Miller

Strengthen Your Core

You've likely seen ads for books or DVDs about strengthening your "core." It sounds like marketing hype, but don't be misled by your natural skepticism. The core is very important to your athletic career. Your body's core is essentially made up of the muscles of your trunk—the area between the shoulder "girdle" and the legs. This includes, of course, your abdominal muscles. Here's why it's so important: Your core is essential to all body movement. Everything you do comes from your core.

Strengthening the core is part of the program for getting stronger and more flexible overall. In fact, you can do most of the core-strengthening exercises in twenty minutes two times a week. Yoga and Pilates are both great for strengthening your core, but the simple pushup is also a great core-strengthening exercise. You can do this at home at your convenience. Boxing, gymnastics, dancing, and basketball are good core-strengthening activities. What's important to know is that time invested in strengthening your core will pay off big time—no matter what sport or workout you prefer.

A WEAK CORE CAN HAMPER THE WAY YOU RUN

When you run with a weak core, your abdominal muscles, which support your spine, sag, and your pelvis does not stay level. You tilt forward into an inefficient running position. Your stride becomes labored and you begin to struggle. A strong core keeps you running efficiently with little or no wasted effort.

"If I ever opened a trampoline store, I don't think I'd call it Trampo-Land, because you might think it was a store for tramps, which is not the impression we are trying to convey with our store. On the other hand, we would not prohibit tramps from browsing, or testing the trampolines, unless a tramp's gyrations seemed to be getting out of control."

—Jack Handy

Get a Trampoline

Bouncing on a trampoline strengthens your legs, increasing their ability to serve as an auxiliary pump for your cardiovascular system, while increasing your pulse for a cardio workout. It also strengthens your voluntary and involuntary muscular system, which helps the entire system work more efficiently and burn more calories. It's also low-impact and spares wear and tear on your joints, feet, knees, and hips. Buy a mini-trampoline to use when you're watching TV. So, if you've got the room in your yard, splurge on a trampoline that you and the kids can enjoy, but if space is limited, a mini-trampoline will give you a workout and there's no reason you can't make it fun, as well.

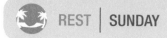
*"Sleep is when all the unsorted stuff comes flying
out as from a dustbin upset in a high wind."*

—William Golding

Try This Recipe for Sweet Dreams

Indigestion can strike at any time of day, but can be especially uncomfortable at night and can lead to painful discomfort, interrupted sleep, and moodiness. Taking a two-step approach to relieving your indigestion may help: 1) Use fruit and vegetable combinations shown to regulate stomach acid and promote more alkaline levels of the digestive tract, and 2) drink chamomile tea before bed. Chamomile tea has been shown to ease indigestion by soothing the esophageal muscles and those of the large and small intestine.

On the uncomfortable nights that indigestion creeps up, turn to your blender for quick relief. This delightfully sweet fruit and veggie combination provides indigestion relief in one sweet treat you can enjoy as dessert or right when the burn hits!

DREAMY DIGESTION

Recipe Yields: 3–4 cups
1 cup romaine lettuce
2 apples, cored and peeled
2 carrots, peeled
1 cucumber, peeled
½ lemon, peeled
2 cups chamomile tea

1. Combine romaine, apples, carrots, cucumber, lemon, and 1 cup of tea in a blender and blend until thoroughly combined.
2. Add remaining 1 cup of tea as needed while blending until desired consistency is achieved.

PER 1 CUP SERVING: Calories 61 | **Fat** 0g | **Protein** 1g | **Sodium** 26mg | **Fiber** 3g | **Carbohydrates** 15g

"In the United States, most of the population consumes about twice as much protein than the human body needs."

—Nathan Brown, martial arts instructor

Bulk Up with Fiber

Nutritionally speaking, fiber is the indigestible part of food you eat—the stuff that passes through your digestive system relatively quickly and intact, such as the bran in grain, the pulp in fruit, and the skin of certain vegetables such as corn. By traveling so quickly, it also rushes other foods through your system, giving cancer-causing compounds less time to do their dirty work, and moving excess calories through your system before they turn into fat, which keeps your metabolic rate high. Fiber also promotes healthy digestion by stimulating the action of beneficial bacteria and dilutes potential carcinogens, reducing their ability to do harm. A diet high in fiber will fill you up so you're less likely to eat unhealthy foods that slow down your metabolism, and it will help you maintain healthy cholesterol and blood sugar levels, making it a great tool for weight management. Studies have shown that consuming between 20 and 30 grams of fiber a day can dramatically reduce your risk for many cancers. Good sources of fiber have at least 2.5 grams of fiber per serving.

Soluble fiber plays two important roles: 1) It binds to bile as it travels through your small intestine, and 2) it helps keep blood sugar levels manageable. Since bile acids assist fat digestion and allow cholesterol to stick around, the faster soluble fiber ushers fat through your system, the less fat and cholesterol you retain. And the steadier your blood sugar levels are, the more efficient your metabolic process remains. Foods containing soluble fiber include:

- Oats/oat bran
- Dried beans and peas
- Nuts
- Barley
- Flaxseed
- Fruits such as oranges and apples
- Vegetables such as carrots
- Psyllium husk

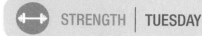

"Muscles need at least forty-eight hours in between
training sessions to recover and repair."

—Shirley S. Archer, fitness professional, Stanford University School of Medicine

Always Rest Between Strength Training Workouts

Strength training works because it places stress on your muscles. This stress causes microscopic injury to your muscle cells. During your rest period, your cells repair this damage. Through repair, your muscles become stronger. If you don't allow your body time to recover, the next time you work out, you'll be placing more stress on already damaged muscle cells. Overtraining slows your progress and can lead to injury. Signs and symptoms of overtraining are decreased performance (you can't lift as much as usual), difficulty in maintaining good form, chronic fatigue, muscle soreness and damage, increased incidence of injuries, joint aches and pains, reduced ability to concentrate, lower self-esteem, increased sensitivity to stress, increased occurrence of illness, decreased rate of healing, and disturbed sleep.

The good news is that rest and recovery time need to be part of your weekly workout schedule. Don't you love it when you can sit on the couch and tell people that it's part of your training program? And, it is. Actually, you're "working in," which is equally important and often neglected. You're allowing the inner process of tissue rebuilding and repair to occur. This is essential to increase your strength and get results.

On the other hand, if you take too much time off between sessions, your muscles will not continue to get stronger without continued stimulation. You will gain new tissue immediately following your last session. But if you spend too much time on the couch, this tissue will atrophy, or shrink.

"Omega-3 fatty acids have so many biological roles because they are a primary element of health for virtually every cell and organ system in the body."

—Andrew Stoll, Faculty, Harvard Medical School

Protect Your Brain by Choosing Fish Low in Mercury Content

Fish is high in omega-3 oils, which is very healthy, but some fish is high in mercury content. Research has shown that nerve cells exposed to mercury caused the formation of neurofibrillar tangles and amyloid plaques, often present in Alzheimer's cases. Dr. Haley, a Canadian researcher, said, "Seven of the characteristic markers that we look for to distinguish Alzheimer's disease can be produced in normal brain tissues, or cultures of neurons, by the addition of extremely low levels of mercury. In addition, research reported in *NeuroReport* has shown that Alzheimer's diseased patients have at least three times higher blood levels of mercury than controls." One particular area of the brain that transmits memories and sensations to higher brain centers contained almost four times as much mercury as did the normal controls. Here's what you need to remember:

- The FDA and EPA recommend limited consumption of shark, swordfish, king mackerel, or tilefish because they contain high levels of mercury.
- The FDA and EPA also recommend no more than 6 ounces (170 g) per week of canned albacore ("white") tuna, tuna steaks, lobster, halibut, and orange roughy. A 6-ounce serving is about the size of two decks of cards or two checkbooks.
- The FDA also recommends that you eat no more than 12 ounces (340 g) per week of fish and shellfish lower in mercury. This equates to two average 6-ounce (170 g) meals.
- Fish lower in mercury include shrimp, canned light tuna (not albacore tuna), salmon, pollock, catfish, cod, crab, flounder/sole, grouper, haddock, herring, mahi-mahi, ocean perch, oysters, rainbow trout, sardines, scallops, tilapia, and trout.

"Before any real benefit can be derived from physical exercises, one must first learn how to breathe properly. Our very life depends on it."

—Joseph Pilates

Learn to Breathe Correctly When Running

One of the most vital yet underrated areas you can work on to improve your running efficiency is correct breathing technique. Since increasing respiration is essential to building endurance, learning how to breathe is essential. The problem is that many people breathe from their chest rather than from their abdominal region while they run. Whether you're a beginner or an experienced runner, take the time to learn and employ the abdominal breathing method. At a minimum, just remember to keep breathing deeply and regularly. In most cases your breathing will take care of itself; as you run faster, you'll breathe faster. And yes, most runners are mouth breathers or at least nose and mouth breathers. It would be impossible to take in adequate oxygen just breathing through your nose.

Your breathing rhythm is very important. Rhythm and stride are closely related to your breathing, whether you take three strides for every breath or two, your breathing and your stride are probably in sync naturally. Beginning runners, though, make the mistake of breathing at a 1:1 rate. This means that they are taking one step while breathing in and one step while breathing out. This is essentially panting, and it is inefficient breathing.

The more economical way to breathe depends, to a large degree, on the pace at which you are running. For your average run, you should breathe 2:2 (taking two steps for every breath in and two steps for every breath out) or 3:3 for longer, slower runs. As you run faster, you may have to breathe more often, which leads to such variations as 2:1 and 1:2 patterns.

*"The mind, when housed within a healthful body,
possesses a glorious sense of power."*

—Joseph Pilates

Embrace Pilates

Pilates is a series of exercises that focus on strengthening core postural muscles to support the spine for correct alignment, an approach used by many hospital rehabilitation programs. Recently, Pilates has become very popular with the general public, particularly those who are looking for a gentle method of increasing core strength, flexibility, and movement.

Pilates is typically taught in health clubs, where private or semiprivate instruction is available on special equipment or group mat classes are conducted without equipment. Pilates uses the resistance of the body to condition and correct itself, with the goal of lengthening and aligning the spine. Like yoga, Pilates offers a low-impact form of strengthening and toning muscles while helping you get more in tune with your body.

The practice focuses on the deep and lateral transverse abdominal muscle, combining stretching and strengthening exercises that target the abdominals, gluteals, and lower-back muscles. It can benefit athletes, those recovering from injuries, and everyone in between.

"I love extreme sports, I like snowboarding and motorcross and rollerblading and hockey."

—Jeremy London

Buy a Pair of Rollerblades and Skate Your Heart Out

Have you tried skating lately? You can still rent skates and get a workout in a roller skating rink or ice skating facility. Ice skating is particularly fun when done in the winter in an outdoor rink. Roller rinks still offer the young and young-at-heart places to get a workout, complete with music and a light show. Another option is to buy some in-line skates designed for skating on paved surfaces such as streets and sidewalks. In-line skates are sleeker and more stable and lightweight than their traditional counterparts. So grab your family or a friend or even your favorite canine for an afternoon outing at the park. Take along a picnic lunch, a bottle of water, and your in-line skates. Don't forget to take along some gloves and wrist-guards to protect your hands and wrists, and pads for your elbows and knees just in case you fall. But don't let the fear of falling keep you from working out and having some fun. Skating particularly works the thighs, calves, and buttocks, and when you see the results on your body for doing that type of regular exercise, you'll exercise your facial muscles, too, into a big smile.

ENJOY THE HEALTH BENEFITS OF SKATING!

If you want to build strong legs, gain balance, and reduce your overall body fat while you get an aerobic workout, pick up a pair of roller skates or in-line skates. A 150-pound person will burn between 400 and 500 calories skating an hour, so if he were to alternate his workouts between skating, cycling, and swimming, he'd burn a significant number of calories during the week and have fun doing it!

"Dogs are our link to paradise. They don't know evil or jealousy or discontent. To sit with a dog on a hillside on a glorious afternoon is to be back in Eden, where doing nothing was not boring—it was peace."

—Milan Kundera

Adopt a Pet

One of the most consistent findings among the many studies evaluating the beneficial role of pets in our lives is that they provide an important measure of stress relief. Simply petting or playing with our favorite pet, whether it's a dog, cat, hamster, or canary, stimulates the production of calming chemicals within the brain and helps us relax. Watching fish in an aquarium has a similar calming effect. The calming influence of small animals is so effective that many doctors recommend daily pet play as therapy for their patients who are under a lot of stress either at work or at home. Fifteen minutes of tossing a yarn ball to some frolicsome kittens is a wonderful and inexpensive way to shed the stress of a hard day at the office. If you're not a cat person, playing fetch with your dog is equally beneficial. The point is to spend time with your pet, whatever the species, and enjoy its company. Talk to it. Pet it. Scratch it behind the ears. Bask in the glow of the pet-owner bond and feel the anxiety melt away. Even the most stressful day is no match for a puppy that's so happy to see you that its tail is a blur.

"Wherever flaxseeds become a regular food item among the people, there will be better health."

—Mahatma Gandhi

Eat More Superfoods

Food is like money. The choices we make in our diet and with our budget can have a profound long-term impact. If you're looking for a great return on your investment, superfoods are the way to go. Superfoods are foods loaded with vitamins, minerals, and other great nutrients that help fight disease, boost metabolism, and make you feel great. All of these foods are unprocessed and reasonably easy to find, so unless you're allergic, go ahead and add them to your diet and enjoy the benefits.

We'll discuss some of these in the coming pages, but some superfoods include:

- Avocado
- Beans
- Blueberries
- Broccoli
- Dark greens
- Flax
- Oats
- Olive oil
- Oranges
- Pomegranate
- Pumpkin
- Salmon
- Soy
- Spinach
- Tea (green or black)
- Tomatoes
- Turkey
- Walnuts
- Yogurt

"Me favorite dish: Popeye spinach kabobs."

—Popeye the Sailor Man

Beef Up with Popeye's Favorite Green Smoothie

When you were a kid, Popeye was one amazing example of what could happen if you ate your spinach! How many times did your parents reference Popeye when trying to get you to eat your spinach? And how often do you reference strength when trying to get your kids to eat greens now? Spinach is packed with vitamins A, B, C, E, and K as well as iron, phosphorous, and fiber. With all of that nutrition delivered in each serving, spinach should be in every athlete's daily diet . . . for strength like Popeye's! This recipe is filled with iron, vitamin K, folate, and fiber, and will have you feeling just as strong.

POPEYE'S FAVORITE

Recipe Yields: 3–4 cups

1 cup spinach
1 kale leaf
1 cup broccoli
3 apples, peeled and cored
2 cups purified water

1. Combine spinach, kale, broccoli, apples, and 1 cup of water in a blender and blend until thoroughly combined.
2. Add remaining 1 cup of water as needed while blending until desired consistency is achieved.

PER 1 CUP SERVING: Calories 76 | **Fat** 0g | **Protein** 2g | **Sodium** 23mg | **Fiber** 3g | **Carbohydrates** 19g

"It's safe to say this [flaxseed] is the most potent plant source of omega-3."

—Elaine Magee, *The Flax Cookbook*

Make It a Good Fat When You Do Eat Fat

Each nerve cell in the brain is surrounded by a protective cell membrane. Receptors for many brain neurotransmitters are found on the membrane. This membrane is composed mostly of different types of fats, which include phosphatidylcholine (PC), also called lecithin; phosphatidylserine (PS); and phosphatidylethanolamine (PE). The function of the nerve cells and the neurotransmitters is highly dependent on the quality of fats that make up the cell membrane and therefore highly dependent on the type of fats and oils in your diet. The makeup of a cell membrane is always in a state of transition; it is constantly influenced by diet, stress, and the immune system.

The bottom line: Your brain needs "good fats" like omega-3 fats, found in certain cold-water fish (bluefish, herring, mackerel, rainbow trout, salmon, sardines, tuna, and whitefish), nuts, avocados, and extra-virgin olive oil, flaxseed oil, peanut oil, and canola oil.

JUST THE FLAX

Flaxseed oil is rich in omega-3s, and has a sweet and nutty flavor. Never use it as a cooking oil, however, as the heat destroys the healthy fats and creates unhealthy free radicals. Instead, add a teaspoonful of flax oil to your favorite salad dressing, or drizzle it over already cooked dishes for your daily quotient of omega-3s. Look for a brand that is cold-pressed and store chilled to keep it fresh.

"Most amateur recreational athletes neglect strength training until they get hurt. Many find out what they should have been doing all along when they end up in physical therapy and are given a set of strength-training exercises. The smart ones keep it up even after the problem is corrected."

—Art Liberman, founder of MarathonTraining.com

Pay Attention to Your Running Technique

As you develop proper running technique, remember the essentials of running mechanics. First, your posture should be guided by a focus on standing erect, imagining a cord coming out of the center and top of your head that gently pulls you straight up. Use your neck muscles to keep your head looking forward, not buried in your chest nor cocked back. Additionally, as you run, keep your face relaxed by letting your jaw drop and your cheeks flap, and keep your eyes looking about 10–20 feet ahead of you.

Concentrating on your body while running, pull up with your abdominal muscles, and focus on running tall with your torso perpendicular to the running surface and your hips directly under your upper body. Let your shoulders hang relaxed and low, not drawn up toward your ears. Hold your arms close to your body, bending them at ninety-degree angles and keeping them near parallel to the ground as they swing counter to your legs. At the same time, hold your hands in a loose fist, with your thumbs up and your palms facing each other.

With a light, efficient, short stride, each foot should land directly under the center of your body weight, not out in front of you. You should land lightly on your heel or ball (midfoot), roll forward onto the ball of your foot, then push off with the balls of your feet and toes in a smooth, fluid, and relatively quiet motion.

"I must be right. Never an aspirin. Never injured a day in my life. The whole country, the whole world, should be doing my exercises. They'd be happier."

—Joseph Pilates

Put Your Toes in the Water with Pilates

Pilates is all about developing strong core muscles by moving your limbs. All you need is a floor mat or yoga mat and about fifteen minutes. When you do each move, pay special attention to the breathing instructions. When you inhale, make it a very slow, deep breath, and feel your body expand with the breath. When you exhale, do it slowly and feel your body get just a little smaller and more relaxed.

Lie with your back on the floor, knees bent, and shins in the air, parallel to the floor. Your lower back should be pressed gently toward the floor, with your arms by your sides and your shoulders away from your ears. Without releasing your abs, slowly drop your right foot toward the floor. You won't be able to get it to the floor, but bring it as far as you can go without losing the contraction in your abs. Bring it back up and repeat with your left foot. Then, try to drop both feet down. They won't go as far as one went. Repeat this whole sequence five times.

ALWAYS KEEP YOUR CORE IN MIND

Try to stay conscious of your core muscles no matter what activity you are doing. To do this, simply tighten, without overly gripping, your abdominal muscles, bringing your lower ribs closer to your hip a fraction. You'll feel a contraction in your abdominals, and that alone will strengthen your core.

"Vice President Cheney is also on vacation. He's in Jackson Hole, Wyoming. What better place for a guy who has had four heart attacks than a place with thin air, rugged hiking, and all-beef dinners? Why don't they get some snow for him to shovel while he's out there, too?"

—Jay Leno

Make Any Vacation an Active One

While adventurous vacations are lots of fun and give you great memories, they can take a lot of planning and money. If you don't have the means or the stamina for such a vacation, don't worry! You can turn almost any vacation into a fitness vacation with just a few easy additions. The following is a list of things you should consider taking with you on your trip, although, of course, the exact list will depend on your location and activity:

- Bathing suit, towel, bathing cap, goggles
- Exercise bands
- Exercise DVDs
- iPod with downloaded workout programs
- Sneakers
- Workout clothes, including bike shorts
- Yoga mat

Finally, if you want to consider luxury with fitness, consider fitness spas! Spas used to be associated with weight loss and deprivation, but now they have accepted and embraced the knowledge that fitness is an essential part of health, weight loss, and relaxation. Spas will encourage you to hike, swim, lift weights, and do Pilates and yoga, and you can do any of these things in Arizona, Tennessee, or Provence!

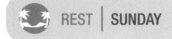

"Within you there is a stillness and a sanctuary to which you can retreat at any time and be yourself."

—Hermann Hesse

Sit Perfectly Still and Do Absolutely Nothing

Zazen is the sitting meditation of Zen Buddhism, but many so-called "Zennists" who don't practice Buddhism practice zazen. Zazen can be accurately defined as "just sitting" and is exactly that—just sitting. It doesn't require any religious or philosophical affiliation. All it requires is the ability to apply the seat of the pants to the floor and stay there for a while. Sounds easy, you say? Hardly. For those of us accustomed to accomplishing something at every moment of the day, just sitting is quite a challenge.

But just sitting accomplishes something amazing if it is practiced every single day for an extended period of time. The mind becomes calmer. The muscles stay more relaxed. Stress fails to get the rise out of your body and your mind that it once did. Suddenly, you hold the reins, not your stress. Suddenly, priorities seem clearer, truths about life, people, and yourself seem more obvious, and things that used to stress you out seem hardly worth consideration anymore.

Just sitting doesn't remove you from the world, however. Choosing not to worry, dwell, and obsess about things means you can concentrate on the real business of living. As your mind opens up, the world opens up, too. All those anxieties suddenly seem like ropes that were tying you down. Just sitting can dissolve the ropes and set you free to really be who you are and live the life you want.

From the Buddhist perspective, zazen is thought to be the path to enlightenment because thousands of years ago the Buddha attained enlightenment while just sitting under a bodhi tree in India. Enlightenment may or may not be your goal. But whatever the case, learning to sit, cultivate stillness and inner silence, and become fully and totally aware of the present moment makes for powerful stress management.

*"There are only ten minutes in the life of
a pear when it is perfect to eat."*

—Ralph Waldo Emerson

Eat Fruit for Multiple Benefits

Fruits offer a multitude of healthy benefits—including being a vitamin-rich (and fiber-rich) way to indulge your sweet tooth. Fruit's sweet flavor comes from fructose, a naturally occurring sugar that serves as a good source of energy—and it's packed with healthy substances such as vitamin C, vitamin A, potassium, folic acid, antioxidants, phytochemicals, and fiber, just to name a few. Citrus fruits, berries, and melons are excellent sources of vitamin C. Dried fruits are available all year long and are an excellent source of many nutrients including fiber. Almost all fruits are good for you, but some are better than others. When it comes to fruit, apples, bananas, berries, citrus fruit, and melons are your best bets because of their high fiber and nutrient content. Researchers at Scripps Clinic found that fruit eaters ate fewer calories overall compared to those not adding fruit to their diet. Fruit can help you satisfy sugar cravings, feel full longer, and eat less.

WEEK FOURTEEN

> **BONUS!**
>
> All fruits contain powerful enzymes that have powerful antibacterial qualities. Enzymes help cleanse the gastrointestinal system by digesting and neutralizing excess protein and fat. If consumed regularly, fruit enzymes can also help flush out the tissues, organs, and muscles by ridding them of these same excesses.

"Strength training includes working with weights, but it is not body building. The objective is not to have massive biceps or washboard abs. You are not aiming for the Arnold Schwarzenegger look. In fact, if you strength train properly, you will probably look leaner than before you started."

—Brent Manley, triathlon veteran

Vary Your Workouts

Many of the benefits of exercise come from the body having to undergo a new experience. When you start walking, running, weight lifting, or doing any other sport, your body gets exposed to new movements and strains. The human body has learned to accommodate to new stresses by adjusting itself to respond to that stress. When you lift weights, your body responds to the stress on your muscles by building more muscle. When you perform cardiovascular exercise, your body responds by the heart building more muscle to accommodate to the need for increased blood flow. Other changes occur as well. In addition to your muscles and heart, other areas of your body also strengthen. Your bones, tendons, and ligaments all restructure to increase their strength. You build more oxygen-carrying red blood cells and oxygen-transporting blood vessels. The body's response to the work of exercise is to make it stronger, and this new strength benefits all aspects of your life.

To improve your overall strength, vary your workouts. If you're lifting weights two days a week, spend two days swimming or three days power walking. The goal is to work different muscle groups and to keep asking your body to do a wider range of exercise.

"Alcohol is a misunderstood vitamin."

—P. G. Wodehouse

Make Sure You're Getting Essential Vitamins

Your brain needs just as many vitamins as the rest of your body does, and it gets them from the bloodstream. When vitamin absorption is reduced or impeded as a result of a poor diet or an illness, the brain is one of the first organs to feel it. Below is a quick rundown of some of the more essential vitamins needed for long-term brain health.

- **Vitamin A.** This antioxidant helps protect brain cells from harmful free radicals and benefits the circulatory system so blood flow to the brain remains strong.
- **Vitamin B$_6$.** This important vitamin helps convert sugar into glucose, which the brain needs for fuel. It also benefits general circulation, which can improve memory.
- **Vitamin B$_1$.** Like B$_{12}$, this nutrient is a potent antioxidant. It is also required for numerous metabolic processes within the brain and peripheral nervous system.
- **Folic Acid.** This nutrient aids cerebral circulation by inhibiting narrowing of the arteries in the neck. Studies also suggest that daily supplements of folic acid can reduce the likelihood of certain age-related psychiatric problems, including dementia.

While you are relatively safe taking a multivitamin, when you want to boost your intake of specific vitamins, it is always wise to run it past your doctor. If you take medication, it is particularly important to make sure elevated levels of vitamins will not adversely affect the medication. Some vitamins can be toxic when taken in huge doses.

ENDURANCE | THURSDAY

"Water consumption is the best method for preactivity or preventative hydration."

—Tina Angelotti, fitness instructor for Krav Maga National Training Center

Stay Hydrated During Endurance Training

Water has a very substantial responsibility within the body. Without water, bodily processes necessary for life would shut down in a matter of days. Water makes up the greatest component of the human body, comprising 50–70 percent of the body's weight. Interestingly, human beings can survive for up to eight weeks without food but only a couple of days without water.

Water has many jobs throughout the body. It acts as a lubricant all over the body—in joints and connective tissues and within organs and vessels—and it even lubricates the body's cells. It also provides electrolytes (sodium, calcium, and magnesium) to the body that are necessary for the balance of fluid compartments found throughout the body. Water also contributes to temperature regulation, helps remove wastes from the body, and can even act as a shock absorber in some parts of the body.

Adults should drink approximately 8 to 12 cups of water per day, maybe more if heavy sweating occurs. If you don't drink enough water your brain will let you know by telling you that you're thirsty. Once you have become thirsty, it usually means you have waited too long to intake water and you may already be dehydrated. It's best to drink water throughout the day to stay properly hydrated.

WHEN ENERGY DRINKS ARE WARRANTED

For exercise that is less than sixty minutes in duration, you should replace the fluid lost from sweat with water. Carbohydrate and electrolyte stores are not usually depleted in this length of time. Anything beyond sixty minutes, carbohydrate and electrolyte replacement does become important and these drinks may be helpful.

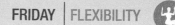

"Patience and persistence are vital qualities in the ultimate successful accomplishment of any worthwhile endeavor."

—Joseph Pilates

Go "Swimming" to Strengthen Your Core

Pilates is all about developing strong core muscles by moving your limbs. All you need is a floor mat or yoga mat and about fifteen minutes. When you do each move, pay special attention to the breathing instructions. When you inhale, make it a very slow, deep breath, and feel your body expand with the breath. When you exhale, do it slowly and feel your body get just a little smaller and more relaxed.

Dive into a Pilates "Swim"

Lie with your stomach on the floor, arms over your head, legs out behind you, and abs gently contracted. Keeping your neck long, lift your arms and legs just a little off the floor and start to "swim" with your arms and legs, fluttering them. Do this about thirty times.

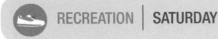

"I do an awful lot of scuba diving. I love to be on the ocean, under the ocean. I live next to the ocean."

—James Cameron

Take Diving Lessons

You've dreamed of seeing coral reefs, sunken treasure ships, and the beautiful world that lies beneath the surface of the ocean. What's keeping you from making your dream a reality? Dive shops often have dive instructors who will teach you the basics in a swimming pool. Then you'll take day trips to the ocean or a body of water where you can put what you've learned to work. Divers watch out for each other and the friendships can continue long after the dive is over. Find the time, money, and the courage to go after your dreams. On the other side of achieving them, you'll feel pleasure and gratification and have a few new friends. And you'll work some muscles and lose lots of weight!

"Leisure time is that five or six hours when you sleep at night."

—George Allen

Get Plenty of Sleep

Your body, including your brain, actually mends and maintains itself when you sleep. If you strength train or do any sort of resistance exercise, then your muscles repair themselves and grow stronger when you're asleep. If you don't sleep, your muscles will stay fatigued and not get stronger. Getting enough sleep helps keep you safe; being sleep-deprived increases the likelihood of accidents and mistakes. It's helpful to first recognize that you want to sleep well, i.e., seven to nine hours of uninterrupted sleep each night. Go to sleep and wake up at the same times. Your body loves regularity. If you are someone who sleeps very late on the weekends and then has trouble waking up for work on Monday, or if you sometimes stay up late and then crash the next evening, you aren't helping yourself. Instead, seek regularity in your sleeping patterns.

TRY A SOOTHING LAVENDER BATH

A warm, lavender-scented bath is a great way to relax and unwind. It also promotes restful sleep. Lavender oil in a hot bath or as a massage oil before bed and lavender oil on the pillow can be very relaxing.

"I'm allergic to chemicals so I eat only organic foods."

—Carol Channing

Eat Organic Foods Whenever Possible

Because organic foods are not subjected to pesticides, they retain more of their natural nutrients and fewer free radicals. This helps maintain cellular health, which in turn helps your body burn foods more efficiently, effectively boosting your metabolism. If you have to economize, opt for organic fruits and vegetables whose skin you eat (apples, pears, peaches, grapes, cherries, peppers, cucumbers, tomatoes, potatoes, green beans), as well as meat, eggs, and milk. Farmers' markets are great resources for organic foods, but you can also look in the phone book or online to find local farms or distributors of organic foods.

When choosing organic produce, look for labels marked "certified" organic. This guarantees that the produce has been grown according to the strict standards set forth by the National Organic Program, including inspection of farms and processing facilities, detailed record keeping, and testing the soil and water for pesticides to ensure government standards are met. Labels reading "transitional organic" mean the food was grown on a farm that has recently converted or is in the process of converting from conventional to organic farming practices.

PESTICIDES AND HERBICIDES ABOUND

Every year, the conventional U.S. agriculture industry goes through more than 1 billion pounds of pesticides and herbicides. Only 2 percent of that actually kills insects; the remaining 98 percent goes into the soil, air, water, and food supply—including the nonorganic fruits and veggies you eat! Buying and consuming organic produce is one way to circumvent this health hazard.

"When I get my heart rate up, I get good exercise and I think it's good for a lot of things, plus it's not hurting my hips right now."

—Mike Ditka

Increase Your Target Heart Rate

As noted in Week Three, your target heart rate is the training zone that is safe and effective for you to improve your cardio respiratory fitness. Now that you're exercising more and building your strength, flexibility, and endurance, it's time to reassess your target heart rate and adjust it upward. Using the formula provided in Week Three, compute your maximum heart rate using the higher figure (65 percent for those who exercise regularly). This would represent a 10 percent increase, which should now be your new goal. Heart rate is an accurate measure of exercise intensity as long as you're a healthy adult. It's easy to estimate your target heart rate.

Let's say you are a forty-year-old woman who is following the suggestions provided and is working hard to get in shape. Your maximum heart rate would be 220 minus 40 (your age), which equals 180. Your beginning heart rate (when you first began following the exercise programs suggested) would have been 55 percent of 180 or 99—likely the point at which you began to sweat and felt strained. However, now that you've bolstered your strength and endurance, upping that to 65 percent of 180 or 117 will provide the boost you need to go to the next level. Remember that you also need to measure your heartbeat: 85 percent of 180 equals 153. You likely began targeting 99 beats per minute, and you should be able to increase that number; however, don't exercise so hard that your heart rate exceeds 153 beats per minute.

And, by the way, congratulations on your progress!

"There's an old saying about those who forget history.
I don't remember it, but it's good."

—Stephen Colbert

Crank Up Your Memory with a Mental Makeover Smoothie

Hate forgetting things? Feel like you have absentmindedness a little too often? This smoothie is designed to get your brain back on track with rich sources of vitamins and minerals that stimulate and rejuvenate brain functions.

BRAIN BOOSTER SMOOTHIE

Recipe Yields: 3–4 cups

1 cup spinach
2 cucumbers, peeled
2 celery stalks
1 tomato
2 cups chamomile tea

1. Combine spinach, cucumbers, celery, tomato, and 1 cup of tea in a blender and blend until thoroughly combined.
2. Add remaining 1 cup of tea as needed while blending until desired consistency is achieved.

PER 1 CUP SERVING: Calories 25 | **Fat** 0g | **Protein** 1g | **Sodium** 29mg | **Fiber** 2g | **Carbohydrates** 5g

---

THE MANY HATS OF SPINACH

In addition to being a rich source of iron and folate (which actually aids in iron absorption), this amazing veggie holds a wealth of vitamins A, B, C, D, and K that provide cancer-fighting power against liver, ovarian, colon, and prostate cancers. By including just 1 cup of this powerful veggie in your daily diet (raw), you can satisfy over 180 percent of your daily value for vitamin K and almost 400 percent of your vitamin A intake!

"American consumers have no problem with carcinogens, but they will not purchase any product, including floor wax, that has fat in it."

—Dave Barry

Make Sure You Consume Good Fats to Fuel Workouts

Fat is an important component to your diet. Many vitamins are "fat soluble," that is, they need fat to be absorbed by your body. Fat also provides long-lasting energy and helps your body produce hormones. In fact, athletes need fat in their diets, preferably two servings a day from fat-rich plant foods. There are many good fats that you should include in your diet. Leading the list is olive oil, a great source of monounsaturated fat, as well as avocados. And don't forget about the good fats in certain nuts (almonds, walnuts, pecans). Certain fish, notably salmon, contain high levels of omega-3 fatty acids, considered very good for the heart. Even butter, a source of saturated fat, has beneficial lauric acid and is believed by many to be superior to margarine, which contains trans fats.

Trans fats, which come from partially hydrogenated oils, are present even in products whose labels declare them to be trans fat free because federal regulations allow that statement if the amount is negligible. Tend to view a product with partially hydrogenated oil as the tenth listed ingredient differently than one with it listed second. There is evidence that no amount of trans fat is healthy in your diet.

Take in fat, but make sure it's the right kind: monounsatured or poly-unsaturated, the kind you get from olive oil, canola oil, and omega-3 fatty acids in fish and leafy green vegetables. Stay away from saturated fat and trans fats.

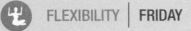
"A few well-designed movements, properly performed in a
balanced sequence, are worth hours of doing sloppy calisthenics
or forced contortion."

—Joseph Pilates

Add Leg Extensions to Improve Overall Flexibility

As with the other Pilates' exercises, everything you do strengthens your core. The stronger your core, the more you are able to execute more complicated exercises, loosen up your joints, and improve your overall flexibility. The following exercise is particularly good for strengthening and limbering up your hips, legs, and hamstrings.

Plank with Leg Extensions

Start in a plank position, which looks like the up position of a pushup. Be sure your torso is long and flat, and your abs are contracted. Your arms are strong, but your elbows aren't locked. Now lift your right leg, toes pointing down. Don't lift your leg too high; it should just go high enough so that you feel a contraction in your butt, but your hips should stay level. Then bend your knee and bring it in toward your chest, once again without changing the line of your hips. Extend your right leg again and then lower your foot to the floor. Repeat on the left side and do this five times on each side.

"It is difficult to realize how great a part of all that is cheerful and delightful in the recollections of our own life is associated with trees."

—Wilson Flagg

Build a Tree House for Your Child and the Child in You

If you've got a tree in your yard strong enough to support a tree house, get the children in your family involved in helping you create the overall design, shopping for the wood and nails, and helping you build it. Not only will your children love you for creating something that will surely give them many pleasurable hours of fun and memories to last throughout their lives, but you'll create a special space to share with them the child in you.

HELP A CHILD DEVELOP A HOBBY

Young children, especially boys, it seems, love to play with cars, trucks, boats, and airplanes. If you've ever watched a seven- to ten-year-old child operating a remote radio-controlled car (also called an RC car), you probably noticed that sooner or later a group has gathered, much to the child's delight, to watch the fancy vehicle maneuvers that he orchestrates through a hand-held controller. Some middle school and high school science teachers have used RC cars as tools for teaching radio-control robotics and programming. Encourage your children to express their interests and develop them into hobbies. You'll enjoy helping them while they are young, and you'll be even happier if, as young adults, they decide to pursue meaningful careers in academic disciplines such as science.

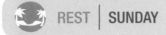

"Tea to the English is really a picnic indoors."

—Alice Walker

Have a Cup of Chamomile Tea

Chamomile tea is widely known for its relaxing properties as well as its apple-like aroma, and is known to soothe the nerves and restore vitality. Contemporary herbalists also recommend chamomile for fever, digestive upsets, anxiety, and insomnia. British researchers recently discovered that chamomile stimulates the immune system's white blood cells. It's particularly recommended for use at the onset of a cold or the flu and its warming and soothing properties promote sleep, the greatest curative of all. Drink a cup or two of tea for relaxation, or at night to promote sleep. Caution: Generally speaking, chamomile is one of the safest herbs available. However, if you are allergic to ragweed or have ever suffered anaphylactic shock, avoid this herb.

"I was a vegetarian until I started leaning toward the sunlight."

—Rita Rudner

Load Up on Leafy Greens

Because greens have very few carbohydrates and a lot of fiber, leafy greens take the body a long time to digest. They fill you up, but they have very few calories and no fat. In fact, most greens have so little impact on blood glucose that many low-carb diets consider them free foods.

Studies show leafy greens pack a powerful nutritional punch by helping reduce heart disease, lung cancer, and colon cancer. A team of researchers from the Harvard School of Public Health found that individuals who consume leafy greens daily had a 23 percent reduction in coronary heart disease. Leafy greens run the gamut in taste, from arugula—which ancient Romans considered an aphrodisiac because of its peppery taste—to iceberg lettuce, which is crunchy and sweet with a very mild flavor. Here are some potent leafy greens and their benefits:

- **Lettuce.** Deep green lettuce is a good source of calcium, chlorophyll, iron, magnesium, potassium, silicon, and vitamins A and E. All types help rebuild hemoglobin, add shine and thickness to hair, and promote hair growth.
- **Parsley.** Packed with chlorophyll, vitamins A and C, calcium, magnesium, phosphorous, potassium, sodium, and sulfur, parsley helps stimulate oxygen metabolism, cell respiration, and regeneration.
- **Spinach, kale, and Swiss chard.** Popeye was right all along. You'll be strong to the finish if you eat your spinach, kale, and chard, which provide ample supplies of iron, phosphorous, fiber, and vitamins A, B, C, E, and K.
- **Watercress.** This delicate leafy green veggie is packed with vitamin C, calcium, and potassium. It also contains acid-forming minerals, which make it ideal for intestinal cleansing and normalizing, and chlorophyll, which stimulates metabolism and circulatory functions.

WEEK SIXTEEN

"Most importantly, a healthy lifestyle is a process. It's a commitment you make to yourself and to those you love and who care for you each and every day."

—Shirley S. Archer, fitness professional, Stanford University School of Medicine

Buy Yourself a Heart Rate Monitor

At some point, if you are serious about building your strength, you will want to get a heart rate monitor. A heart monitor is essential for accurately managing your efforts to achieve certain goals or managing the balance between aerobic and anaerobic conditioning, fat loss, or cardio threshold conditioning. Only with a heart monitor can you know for sure that you have worked out at an intensity level appropriate to your goals. With monitors readily available and inexpensive, there is no reason anyone should not use one.

There are many heart rate monitors on the market. Some simply tell you your current heart rate, while others allow you to connect to your computer so you can record and download your heart rate and give you a summary for each training period. Some monitors will even allow you to set the type of workout you are going to do and then warn you when you are above or below your target heart rate. Prices range from $29 to over $500.

Once you know your heart rate, you can train in specific zones tailored to your goals for that training period. Each zone corresponds to a heart rate range relative to your maximum heart rate. Aerobic conditioning, which strengthens your heart and lungs, takes place when training keeps your heart rate between 70 percent and 80 percent of your max heart rate. Anaerobic conditioning, which improves your ability to perform very intensely for short periods of time, takes place when training keeps your heart rate between 80 percent and 90 percent of your max heart rate. Training above 90 percent of your maximum heart rate can only be maintained for short periods of time.

"A good puzzle, it's a fair thing. Nobody is lying. It's very clear, and the problem depends just on you."

—Erno Rubik

Tease Your Brain with Word Ladders

Link these word pairs together with a ladder of words. Each step in the ladder must be a real word and must differ from the previous word by only one letter. For example, CAT can be linked to DOG with these steps: CAT, COT, DOT, DOG. There are many possible solutions for these puzzles, but try to use only the given number of steps:

EGG TO HEN (ten steps)

_____   _____

TIME to BELL (five steps)

_____   _____

SING to TONE (five steps)

_____   _____

"To make a muscle grow, you must force it to go beyond its capabilities. The most potent way to apply that force is to train to failure. Training to failure means . . . the muscles are forced to grow stronger and bigger."

—Nasser El Sonbaty

Add More Reps to Your Weight-Lifting Routine to Bolster Endurance

The intensity of your weight training relates to your effort level. This is based on training volume. The volume of your training is measured by repetitions, sets, and resistance. All strength-training exercises are defined by these factors. A moderate program consists of eight to ten exercises that include the following major muscle groups:

- **Chest:** pectoral muscles
- **Shoulders:** deltoid muscles, rotator cuff, scapular stabilizers, trapezius
- **Arms:** biceps, triceps, forearm
- **Back:** latissimus dorsi, erector spinae, trapezius
- **Abdomen:** rectus abdominis, obliques, transversus
- **Legs:** gluteals, quadriceps, hamstrings, calves

When it comes to counting reps to muscle failure, lifting a very heavy weight that can only be lifted a few times would be considered high-intensity training. Very heavy lifting is only appropriate for athletes and experienced exercisers. Athletes perform very heavy lifting to produce strength and power gains.

For most people, a moderate intensity approach minimizes injury and produces results. Performing eight to twelve repetitions to muscular failure is considered moderate intensity. By performing between eight to twelve repetitions, you strike a balance between building muscle strength and endurance.

When you select your level of weight for each exercise, make sure that you are feeling challenged, but not overwhelmed. If you can perform 15 repetitions of an exercise easily, that's a sign that your weight is too light. If you can't do 8 reps, then the weight is too heavy. Always start light and increase weight in the smallest possible increments. Don't try to force a lift. You may injure yourself.

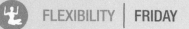

"In 10 sessions, you will feel the difference. In 20, you will see the difference. And in 30, you'll be on your way to having a whole new body."

—Joseph Pilates

Increase the Intensity of Your Plank Exercises

Now that you've mastered several Pilates exercises, it's time to rev up your Pilates workout. When you do each move, pay special attention to the breathing instructions. When you inhale, make it a very slow, deep breath, and feel your body expand with the breath. When you exhale, do it slowly and feel your body get just a little smaller and more relaxed.

Side Plank

This is an isometric exercise, which means you just hold the pose, rather than moving through it. It's tough, so here are three variations to try:

- Hard Side Plank: Put your right leg and your right elbow on the floor, keeping your left leg long, with your left foot on the floor, and your torso straight and long. Your left arm can be down along your side. Hold this position for two to five breaths.
- Harder Side Plank: Do the same position above, but balance on your right bent leg and your right hand. Hold for two to five breaths.
- Hardest Side Plank: Start in the plank position. Now, bring the right palm toward your left palm so it's on the floor just below the center of your chest. Now turn your body as you bring the outside of your right foot on the floor in line with the palm. Stack the left foot on top of the right, with the inner edges of the feet in contact. Press the right hand down into the floor and lift the hips, making the legs and torso one straight line. Lift the left arm toward the ceiling, making the arms one straight line. Breathe and hold for two to five breaths. Come back to the plank position and repeat on the left.

"I'm not going to vacuum until Sears makes one you can ride on."

—Roseanne Barr

Spend the Day Cleaning Your House

Now, this is a funny thing. These days, many people think of house-cleaning as beneath them, even though they are proud of their clean homes. In other words, as with gardening, they let someone else do the work. And that's a shame, because housecleaning is, in many ways, the perfect cross-training workout. It combines cardio (especially if you're scrubbing bathrooms or floors), resistance training in your upper body, and flexibility (because you are moving around a lot and constantly changing position). In many ways, housecleaning is like dancing—it's constant motion. And cleaning your house yourself will save you money!

Another very effective strategy is to clean your house in 10-minute, 20-minute, or 30-minute breaks in the evening, especially if the TV is usually on. Get up during commercials and wash your sinks, or turn off the TV during that half-hour show you don't really like and do the whole bathroom. Not only will you burn a nice number of calories, but the energy blast will lighten your mood and you'll be happy with the reward of a cleaner house.

EXACTLY HOW IS THIS RECREATION?

If you think of recreation as a way to get physical exercise, clean-ing house offers a variety of activities that can make a change in your body, including your heart and muscles: vacuuming, dust-ing, washing floors, scrubbing bathrooms, and washing win-dows. Because of differences in body size, activities, and energy output, no one knows exactly how many calories you'll burn, but rough estimates are anywhere from 100 to 300 calories per hour, depending on your intensity level.

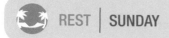

"Too many people spend money they haven't earned, to buy things they don't want, to impress people they don't like."

—Will Rogers

Give Your Credit Card a Rest: Go on a Buying Strike

Whether or not you use a credit card to buy goods, refraining from mindlessly participating in consumerism would probably do your spirit a lot of good—and it would be a great habit to embrace. Start today by designating one day in the week ahead to absolutely not put one foot in a store or go online to shop. No gas, no food, no latte on the way to work. *Nada.* Save your dough and enjoy the bounty of the planet and the blessings of family and friends.

Once you try it, and discover how freeing it can be to focus on savoring the free things in life rather than blindly or habitually consuming, you may want to go on a buying strike two days a week. And even if you only stick to one day a week (or one a month), bringing your spending habits to consciousness will make you a fully conscious, and thus smarter, consumer.

Other ways to be a conscious consumer:

- **Support socially conscious businesses.** Seek out and support retailers who take care of the environment and treat employees and customers fairly.
- **Support your local small businesses, as they need your support far more than multinational corporations.** It also helps your local economy and offers you a chance to get to know business owners who are members of your community.
- **Boycott unethical businesses.** Refuse to conduct business with those that engage in immoral practices such as using offshore child labor, exploiting workers through low wages and putting them in harm's way, or forcing them to live in hazardous housing.

"Nothing says holidays, like a cheese log."

—Ellen DeGeneres

Satisfy a Craving Healthfully

When your body (or your mind) seems to be screaming for ice cream, there are ways to offer up a sweet, creamy dessert that is far lower in calories and whose high protein content will actually fill you up! Fat-free ricotta cheese, for example, won't wreak havoc with your caloric or fat intake, and will provide the taste and feel of fat and a healthy dose of protein. Here's a simple recipe that can be whipped up whenever a craving strikes:

SWEET RICOTTA DESSERT

Serves 1
¼ cup fat-free ricotta cheese
½ teaspoon vanilla extract
1 teaspoon Splenda

Combine ingredients in a bowl, stir well, and enjoy!

PER SERVING: Calories 51 | Fat 0g | **Protein** 9g | **Sodium** 120mg | **Fiber** 0g | **Carbohydrates** 4g

---

SO WHAT IS RICOTTA CHEESE?

It's an Italian cheese produced from whey, the limpid, low-fat, nutritious liquid that gets separated out from the curd when they make cheese. Ricotta has a grainy texture, looks creamy white, and tastes slightly sweet. The cheese contains around 5 percent fat and has a texture that is quite similar to some of the variants of cottage cheese, though it is considerably lighter.

"I also get fed up with the fact that casting agents and directors have this impression of me as being frail and petite. I find it very patronizing. I'm quite beefy and strong. I was a gymnast in school and I have lots of muscles."

—Helena Bonham Carter

Choose Exercises That Strengthen Your Core Muscles

Your core muscles are the abdominal muscles that do the heavy lifting in your life. Strengthening your core muscles is essential to building a strong muscular system, which also improves your ability to burn calories quicker and more efficiently. The abdominals are comprised of the rectus abdominus, the obliques, and the transverse abdominus. The rectus abdominus runs from your rib cage past your belly button, down into your pubic crest. This muscle can be contracted by bringing your hips closer to your rib cage, as you do in regular crunches. The external and internal obliques run in a more diagonal pattern and are located on each side of the rectus abdominus. The obliques are responsible for trunk rotation (twisting) and lateral bending. The transverse abdominus is the deepest abdominal muscle. It is commonly referred to as a stabilizing belt for your trunk and spine. This muscle is not responsible for movement, but it is a vital component to lower back health. These muscles combine with those of the lower back to form what is commonly referred to as the core.

Activities like martial arts, dancing, soccer, gymnastics, swimming, boxing, and basketball all require you to engage your core regularly. All of these options force you to twist and bend at the waist a lot, which is great work for your core muscles. The elliptical machine and the stationary bicycle do not do as much to strengthen your core. When you plan out your exercise regime, make sure you include abdominal strength-training exercises for five to twenty minutes every other day. Your mission is to choose a variety of exercises that work each core muscle in a challenging way. Start slowly and progress to extremely challenging exercises.

"Fish oil has been shown in a series of studies by Andrew Stoll at Harvard to ease the symptoms of bipolar disorder and depression."

—Charles Barber, author of *Comfortably Numb*

Take Fish Oil Capsules

Over the years, fish oil has been touted to help with a myriad of medical problems—including protecting the body from the onset of Parkinson's and schizophrenia—but what is very exciting is its ability (because of the high levels of omega-3 it contains) to lower the body's cholesterol levels, reduce overall blood pressure, and keep you full for longer. There is also recent evidence from the *International Journal of Obesity* that suggests fish oil helps with the body's ability to burn fat and that those who supplement with fish oil will metabolize more fat as they exercise. When you're looking for a fish oil supplement, reach for those containing 300 milligrams of the fatty acid EPA and 200 milligrams of the fatty acid DHA and take two each day. If you have an increased risk of bleeding, ask your doctor before taking omega-3 supplements.

"Bodybuilding is much like any other sport. To be successful, you must dedicate yourself 100 percent to your training, diet, and mental approach."

—Arnold Schwarzenegger

Go Slow and Steady When Lifting Weights

When you perform a movement, move with control. People who are new to weight training often use momentum to move weights. Using momentum results from building up speed by swinging your weights. Because an object in motion tends to remain in motion unless acted on by an external force, the use of speed requires less muscle control. It also makes it easier. Weight training is one of those activities where you need to pay attention so you force yourself to keep it challenging.

Focus on your goal for weight training. You're not weight training to win a prize for the number of pounds that you lift. Weight training is more process oriented. The specific number of pounds that you lift is not important. You get stronger over time. What's important is that you are able to execute your exercises in a slow and controlled manner with good posture. This is how you will improve your strength.

When you use your muscles and not momentum, you should be able to lower the weight and lift it with control. Since many movements are assisted by gravity on the way down, slow movements challenge your muscles. If you simply drop weights on the way down, you risk hurting yourself or damaging equipment—and it's painful on the eardrums.

Fast, jerky movements mean you're not maximizing your training benefits. Every minute you spend training should count. Perfect practice leads to perfect results. Take your time. Remember why you are training. Move with control. Execute your exercises smoothly through a full range of motion. Over time, you'll notice a huge difference in your body awareness and ability to control your movements.

*"Not only is health a normal condition, but it is our
duty not only to attain it but to maintain it."*

—Joseph Pilates

Use an Exercise Ball and Pilates to Strengthen Your Core

Just sitting on an exercise ball challenges your core because you have to stabilize your torso muscles in order to not roll off. These Pilates exercises, even when they aren't focusing on your core muscles, are challenging because you have to keep your balance as you do them.

Lean Back with Open Arms

Sit on an exercise ball, butt slightly forward from the top, knees bent, feet on the floor. Contract your abs, and keep your shoulders away from your ears as you bring your arms up in front of you to shoulder height in a circle, fingers close together, and lean back slightly. Now, turn to your right as you open your right arm out to the side and behind you. Come back to center and repeat to the left without sitting up. Come back to the center. Repeat the sequence five times on each side.

*"I always thought a yard was three feet, then
I started mowing the lawn."*

—C. E. Cowman

Spend the Day Working in Your Yard

Years ago, only wealthy people employed gardeners and landscapers, but today gardeners and landscapers work for everyone in the neighborhood, even in middle-class neighborhoods. And what are the owners—and kids—in these middle-class homes doing while someone else is raking their leaves? Often, watching TV, eating, or surfing the Internet.

And that's a shame, because digging, raking, and planting are moderate-intensity activities, equivalent to taking a brisk walk. Even better? Tough gardening chores such as mowing the lawn with a push mower, chopping wood, and shoveling are comparable to skiing or playing doubles tennis. These activities do not replace true exercise routines, but they are a perfect way to reverse the curse of inactivity.

Working in your yard offers one more important benefit: It is psychologically uplifting. Being outside, pruning your hedges or mowing your lawn is time spent interacting with nature. If you engage your whole family, all of you will be able to quickly see the fruits of your labors and you can treat yourselves to a cup of frozen yogurt afterward.

DO NO HARM

To make gardening safer, remember that when you're weeding, bend at the knees rather than at the waist. Also, try to alternate your grip when using tools. Additionally, don't do too much. You shouldn't work longer in your garden than you would take a walk, for example. Finally, stretch when you need to and don't sit in one position for too long.

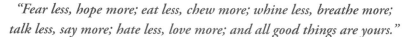
"Fear less, hope more; eat less, chew more; whine less, breathe more; talk less, say more; hate less, love more; and all good things are yours."

—Swedish Proverb

Practice Deep Breathing to Relax

Deep, mindful breathing exercises are a great way to trigger your body's relaxation response. Plus, they are easy to learn, fast to perform, and require no equipment. The following breathing exercise will help you ease tensions and restore your sense of balance and calm—and do the health of your body, mind, and spirit a world of good. As you emerge from your restorative relaxation time, remind yourself that you have the power to create your own health and to enjoy all that life has to offer to you.

Sit or lie down in a safe and comfortable spot with no distractions. Loosen any tight clothing; unbutton or untie anything that is restrictive on your body. Begin to breathe consciously, following your breath in and out of your lungs. Breathe in through the nostrils, out through the mouth. Pay full attention to your breath, in and out, in and out. Listen to the sound and feel the rhythmic pulsing of it. Continue this until you begin to feel calm and relaxed, a state usually signaled by your breath becoming slow and even.

Add Visualization to Deepen Your Relaxation

You can deepen your relaxation using breath by imagining that you are breathing in the positive vital force of life, and exhaling all tension and negative feeling or experience. One way to do this is to choose two colors, one for the positive and one for the negative energy: See a stream of one color (positive) coming into your body as you inhale, and a stream of the other color (negative) flowing out of your body as you exhale. The colors white and black are easy to identify—white is the pure energy of light, and black represents any dark thoughts. But feel free to use any color that represents healing energy and release of negative energy to you. Don't worry if distracting thoughts arise. Let them float off like soap bubbles in the air and return to attending to your breathing.

"I am convinced digestion is the great secret to life."

—Sydney Smith

Make It a Curry Day

One of the primary ingredients in curry, turmeric, aids digestion by stimulating the flow of bile and the breakdown of dietary fats. Curry is a powerful source of antioxidants, containing within a single teaspoon as many antioxidants as in a half cup of grapes. Its antioxidant and anti-inflammatory capabilities can be traced back to curcumin, which gives turmeric its characteristic yellow color. For centuries, curcumin alone has been used to cure everything from heartburn to arthritis and, according to *Earl Mindell's Herb Bible,* "the herbs that are combined to make curry help prevent heart disease and stroke by reducing cholesterol and preventing clots." Here's a tasty recipe to try:

SPICY CURRY SESAME CHICKEN

Serves 6
6 boneless, skinless chicken breasts, in chunks
½ cup chicken broth
1 teaspoon cornstarch
1 tablespoon curry powder
½ teaspoon all-purpose seasoning
1 clove fresh garlic, minced
1 teaspoon sesame seeds
1 cup sliced yellow onions
1 tablespoon olive oil
2 tablespoons hot sauce

1. Spray large skillet with nonstick spray.
2. Mix all ingredients in a large bowl. Pour mixture into skillet. Cook on medium high for 10 to 12 minutes, stirring often. Simmer for 5 to 10 minutes. Serve with brown rice, rice noodles, or another healthy grain.

PER SERVING: Calories 169 | **Fat** 4g | **Protein** 28g | **Sodium** 286mg | **Fiber** 1g | **Carbohydrates** 3g

WEEK EIGHTEEN

"A warm-up does more than just prepare your muscles for a workout. Warming up should be seen holistically as a way to bring your muscles, cardiovascular system, and the rest of your body (as well as your mind) to a state of readiness for your workout."

—Jeff Levine, Krav Maga instructor

Match Your Warm-Up Time to Your Workout Time

A proper warm-up increases your cardiorespiratory system's ability to do work. It also makes your body more efficient in the amount of oxygen that it is able to absorb and utilize. This increased efficiency improves the flow of blood to your heart, which reduces your risk of suffering exercise-induced cardiac abnormalities. It also causes your body's temperature to rise, thus reducing your risk for experiencing the many exercise-related injuries that can be inflicted upon a "cold" muscle structure.

The amount of time you spend on your warm-up should be based upon the length and intensity of your workout. For example, a fifteen-minute warm-up is sufficient for an hour-long workout at a level of moderate to high intensity. However, a workout of two to four hours in length, within that same intensity range, would need a warm-up of between thirty minutes to an hour.

GET YOUR MINDSET ON

Athletes and competitors at all levels of competition, from recreational to Olympic caliber, often feel that practicing some sort of skill-related activity before competing in an event helps to mentally prepare them. Such mental preparation helps them to perform better at the moment of truth. Whether you are training for a specific athletic event or just getting ready for a jog, mentally preparing yourself to train is essential in achieving a positive state of mind.

*"The demon of intemperance ever seems to have delighted
in sucking the blood of genius and generosity."*

—Abraham Lincoln

Minimize Alcohol Consumption

Watch out for alcohol and other mind-numbing drugs. Most experts agree that a drink a day won't threaten your health, but abuse of alcohol or recreational drugs can diminish your ability to absorb stimuli from the world around you and result in a limited ability to form new memories. Brain scans of alcoholics tend to show low activity in the cerebellum, the brain's major coordination center. Alcohol should be consumed in moderation—preferably one drink every few days and a maximum of one or two glasses a day. Because it is considered a neurotoxin, more than two glasses of alcohol a day can adversely affect your health. Also, it's a harsh but true fact: Alcohol shrinks your brain. If you value your brain cells, limit alcohol consumption.

YOUR BRAIN ON ALCOHOL

Clearly, alcohol affects your brain, even in the short term. The long-term effects of too much alcohol consumption on the brain are much worse, and include:

- Blackouts
- Permanent memory lapses
- Nerve damage
- Brain shrinkage
- Vitamin B_1 (thiamine) deficiency
- Alterations in the balance of neurotransmitters such as GABA

Serious alcohol consumption on a regular basis can also lead to several debilitating brain disorders.

"The last three or four reps is what makes the muscle grow. This area of pain divides the champion from someone else who is not a champion. That's what most people lack, having the guts to go on and just say they'll go through the pain no matter what happens."

—Arnold Schwarzenegger

When You're Ready to Progress, Increase Your Reps

As you start feeling stronger, you may be tempted to quickly increase your weight loads. Resist the temptation. Before you increase the weight level, increase the number of your repetitions. If you're performing all twelve of your repetitions with good form, then bump up your weight. The rule of thumb is to increase your weight by roughly five percent. Listen to your body. Let your muscles be the judge. You don't want to increase your weight levels so much that you injure yourself or experience excessive muscle soreness.

Add a conservative amount of weight and see how it feels. Trust your body. If it feels within a comfortable range for you, it's likely to be a good increment. If it feels like too much, it probably is. You also want to change your exercises to challenge your muscles in different ways. Muscles need variety. Keep stimulating them. Your mind will also appreciate the change. If your program feels boring to you, your body is probably bored, too. Time for a change.

"I work out, I go to Pilates, I walk, and I eat everything I can get my hands on."

—Sally Kellerman

Combine Leg Exercises with an Exercise Ball to Strengthen Your Core

Here are two more Pilates exercises using an exercise ball that will strengthen your core.

Single Leg Stretch

Lie on your back with the ball in your hands, above your torso. Press your lower back gently into the floor as you raise your legs to a 45-degree angle from your hips. Keeping your shoulders away from your ears, raise your head, neck, and shoulders off the floor. Bend your right knee and bring it in toward your chest. The ball should be just above your knee. Hold this position for two counts, then switch legs without moving your upper body and hips. Do this eight times on each leg.

Criss Cross

Lie on your back with the ball in your hands, above your torso. Press your lower back gently into the floor as you raise your legs to a 45-degree angle from your hips. Keeping your shoulders away from your ears, raise your head, neck, and shoulders off the floor. Bend your right knee and bring it in toward your chest. As you do this, twist toward your left slightly, bringing your hand and the ball down toward your left knee. Hold this position for two counts, come back to the start position, and then go to the other side. Do this eight times on each leg.

"I do the cooking at home. Where we eat no more than 100 grams of meat a day and have 'tons' of fresh vegetables. I prepare the vegetables with a wide range of herbs, spices and such. We also keep on hand lots of fruit, yogurt and great breads."

—Graham Kerr

Design and Plant an Herb Garden

Gardening gives you the opportunity to work out in the fresh air. And nothing beats fresh-picked herbs when you want to intensify the taste of salsas, sauces, and savory dishes. Using a spade to turn over dirt and dig in fertilizers and soil amendments can give you a workout. The number of calories burned while gardening, according to a variety of Internet sites about fitness, ranges between 250 and 272 per hour. That's roughly one Starbucks grande Caffè Latte made with milk, or one Snickers bar. You can get a bit more of a workout if you use heavy equipment during your time in the garden, for example, a rototiller or cutting trees with a chain saw. The calories then add up to around 400 to 405 per hour. But if you love to cook and also appreciate having fresh herbs as well as fruits and vegetables packed with vitamins, minerals, and other nutrients, consider designing and planting a garden and then combine the gardening with cooking for a healthier you.

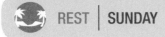

"Plants that wake when others sleep. Timid jasmine buds that keep their fragrance to themselves all day, but when the sunlight dies away let the delicious secret out to every breeze that roams about."

—Thomas Moore

Light an Aromatic Candle

Smell is the most potent of all the senses because the information is delivered straight to your hypothalamus. As moods, motivation, and creativity all stem from the hypothalamus, odors affect all of these processes. Think of a disgusting odor and how it can affect your appetite— or think of a fragrance that brings back a pleasant memory of a loved one, and you'll get the idea of how intimately intertwined scents are with our emotions, memories, and ideas. Light a candle whose fragrance invokes pleasant memories, lie back, and soothe your hypothalamus. Choose whatever scent pleases you, or research online for scents that are associated with relaxation.

"Every man is the builder of a Temple called his body,
nor can he get off by hammering marble instead."

—Henry David Thoreau

Lose 10 Percent of Your Excess Body Weight

Did you know that men with waistline circumferences over 40 inches and women with waists greater than 35 inches have a significantly greater risk of a heart attack than their slimmer pals? Did you also know that by losing just 5 to 10 percent of your excess body weight, you can lower your blood pressure, cholesterol, insulin, and triglyceride levels? Losing weight shouldn't be just about looking good; it offers major health advantages. Use this knowledge to create a nutritious, metabolism-boosting diet. Follow it with vigor and determination, and you'll not only whittle your waist, you'll whittle your hips, thighs, arms, and everything else!

WEEK NINETEEN

"This [warm-up] is your time to get your blood pumping and work up a light sweat. Starting out at a high-level intensity or difficulty will completely defeat the entire purpose of doing a warm-up in the first place."

—Nathan Brown, martial arts instructor

Try Calisthenics as a Way to Warm Up for a Workout

Warm-ups are usually classified as either general or specific. However, there is a lot of overlap between the two. One type of warm-up is not necessarily better than the other type—they are both of equal importance. Most warm-ups have both general and specific movements throughout. If you focus too much on either type of warm-up, you will miss out on the benefits of the other. You should try to achieve a balance between both general and specific warm-ups in your routine to achieve a balanced and evenly prepared body that will give you maximum benefits.

A specific warm-up contains movements that mimic the activity or anticipated movements or exercises that are about to follow your warm-up routine. A specific type of warm-up is a lot like rehearsing a particular skill a few times before doing it at full speed or power.

A general warm-up employs movements that are not necessarily related to the movements and exercises of the workout routine that is about to follow. This type of warm-up includes calisthenics, and any other kinds of general body movements that make you feel loosened up. Jumping jacks, squats, lunges, pushups, and sit-ups are all good examples of calisthenic-type warm-up exercises. When performed at a low- to medium-range impact level, these exercises are great to use in a general warm-up. Remember, this is your warm-up not your workout, so don't overdo it. These exercises are meant to prepare your body for your preworkout stretch and workout.

"Meet me down in the bar! We'll drink breakfast together."

—W. C. Fields

Restore Your Brain with a Green Bloody Mary

The alcoholic Bloody Mary may be tempting, but the alcohol can do a load of damage to your cells, skin, digestion, and your brain. This nonalcoholic green version of the Bloody Mary has all of the necessary ingredients to repair exactly what the alcoholic version destroys!

THE GREEN BLOODY MARY

Recipe Yields: 3–4 cups

1 cup watercress
2 tomatoes
2 celery stalks
½ lemon, peeled
1 tablespoon horseradish
½ teaspoon cayenne pepper (optional)
1 cup purified water

1. Combine watercress, tomatoes, celery, lemon, horseradish, and cayenne with ½ cup purified water in a blender and blend until thoroughly combined.
2. Add remaining ½ cup water while blending until desired texture is achieved.

PER 1 CUP SERVING: Calories 19 | **Fat** 0g | **Protein** 1g | **Sodium** 36mg | **Fiber** 1g | **Carbohydrates** 4g

*"My feeling is that any day I am too busy to run
is a day that I am too busy."*

—John Bryant

Run First, Lift Later

Combining running and weight lifting is a great way to build your endurance—and your strength. If you are doing both on the same day, runners should ideally run first and do strength training second, preferably not back-to-back. The best thing to do is schedule several hours between a run and your strength workout. You may run in the morning and then do your strength routine at lunchtime or in the evening. If you are forced to perform the two routines together, do your run first and then your strength training. If you're doing a long run or a speed workout, hold off on the strength training afterward. You'll probably be too tired to perform it properly.

Some have recommended that you perform your hard running and strength training on the same day (but separate the two), followed by an easy run the next day so you have time to recover. Experiment to see what feels right to you. You might find it easier to do your strength training on a light running day or even on a rest day. For more advanced runners, if you do strength training on a rest day, go very easy on the legs or skip the leg workouts entirely if you will be racing or doing a speed work session the next day.

"I tried yoga once but took off for the mall halfway through class,
as I had a sudden craving for a soft pretzel and world peace."

—Terri Guillemets

Boost Your Omegas with a Tasty Smoothie

Omega-3s are vital to your body's ability to stay agile. In this tasty recipe, omega-3s are plentiful without the need for salmon or rich meats. If salmon isn't your favorite food, consider smoothies that contain flax for your daily value of omegas.

OH, MY! OMEGAS

Recipe Yields: 3–4 cups
1 cup watercress
½ cantaloupe, rind and seeds removed
1 banana, peeled
1 orange, peeled
1 cup raspberries
1 tablespoon flax seeds
2 cups purified water

1. Combine watercress, cantaloupe, banana, orange, raspberries, flax seeds, and 1 cup of water in a blender and blend until thoroughly combined.
2. Add remaining 1 cup of water as needed while blending until desired consistency is achieved.

PER 1 CUP SERVING: Calories 102 | **Fat** 2g | **Protein** 2g | **Sodium** 18mg | **Fiber** 5g | **Carbohydrates** 23g

"Music is your own experience, your thoughts, your wisdom.
If you don't live it, it won't come out of your horn."

—Charlie Parker

Attend a Music Camp

What would summer be without music camps? Do you love to play the saxophone? Keyboards? Electric violin or guitar or drums? How about singing for the opera or musicals? Check out music camps offered in your region of the country. They aren't just for kids anymore. Some focus on a single instrument. Others are geared toward chamber orchestra or band music. If you are a beginner, there are camps for adults who are just beginning to think about music for themselves. Some camps are associated with competitions. Many offer scholarships if you can't afford to attend. To find one that is right for you, search for "adult beginner music camp." Nurture your aspiration to learn music because it will be a source of joy throughout your life.

BONUS: IT'S FABULOUS FOR YOUR BRAIN

Reading music and playing an instrument has consistently been shown to morph your brain in ways that few other activities can. If you're already a musician, learn to play a new instrument, or take up songwriting, composing, or producing. You get the drift . . . challenge your mind and your coordination by doing something you've never done before, something that makes you—and your brain—grow.

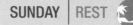

*"Follow Descartes! Do not give up the religion of your youth
until you get a better one."*

—Martin H. Fischer

Attend at Least One Religious Service This Week

Even in our materialistic, consumer-driven society, you can live a purposeful, self-actualized, meaningful, and happy life. Research suggests that participation and belief in a religious faith or spiritual tradition is an important ingredient for having that kind of life. One way to stay in touch with your core spiritual beliefs is to regularly attend a religious service or a gathering in which your faith and belief is shared. Some studies link such regular participation to a greater sense of well-being, a stronger connection to community, reinforcement of your beliefs, and a more stable, healthier, and happier family life. If you don't have a specific faith, create a regular ritual to honor what you believe in. It can be an elaborate affair or as simple as finding a few minutes to read about or reflect upon beliefs you find inspiring.

DESIGNATE ONE CORNER OF YOUR HOME AS SACRED SPACE

Create an area in your home that can serve as a sanctuary for yoga, prayer, writing in your journal, sipping tea, reading, and reflecting. Make your sacred space private. Add a screen, a large plant, a curtain, or something that defines and separates that space from the rest of the house. Add a small table to hold your spiritual texts, sacred objects, candles, incense, holy oil, or prayer beads. A window or door with a view of a lake or garden is an added bonus. Otherwise hang a piece of silk, a batik, or spiritual art. Regularly retreat to your sanctuary to reconnect with your own inner joy.

"All happiness depends on a leisurely breakfast."

—John Gunther

Eat a High-Fiber Breakfast to Lower Fat Consumption

If you think breakfasts are unhealthy, maybe you need to rethink what you're eating. A doughnut and coffee aren't going to start your day off right, but what about eggs, whole-wheat toast, and a small salad or piece of fruit? By eating a high-fiber breakfast, you can stay fuller for longer, and it will help you not reach for that sugary snack in the office kitchen or in the pantry. Research has shown that eating a high-fiber, low-fat breakfast can result in a lower fat intake for the entire day, which helps your metabolism because it can use the fat already stored in your body for energy. If you can't stand the thought of eating breakfast, start out with something like toast or fruit and bring a snack with you for later in the morning when you get hungry.

Here are some healthy suggestions to enjoy in the morning:

- Fiber-rich, cold cereal with fruit and skim milk
- Bran muffin and a banana
- Hard-boiled egg, grapefruit juice, whole-grain toast
- Yogurt with fruit or low-fat granola cereal
- Peanut butter on whole-wheat toast and an orange
- Oatmeal with raisins or berries
- Breakfast smoothie (blend fruit and skim milk)

"Approximately 50 percent of American adults cannot even carry a ten-pound bag of groceries."

—The National Center for Health

Match Your Warm-Up Exercises to Your Fitness Level

Your warm-up should begin with some easy cardiorespiratory exercises that are both simple and gradual. It should be sufficient enough to increase your muscle and core temperatures without causing you to experience fatigue or a reduction in your energy stores. This means you should take your time with your first few exercises. By the end of your warm-up you should feel energized and ready to pick up your intensity level rather than feeling as if your warm-up was strenuous enough to be your entire workout.

This makes your warm-up highly individualized. For a normally sedentary person, this may mean walking briskly for five minutes; while someone with more exercise experience may need to jog for five minutes. Any exercise that increases your heart rate and respiratory rate will work. Cycling, elliptical machines, treadmills, and stair masters are considered cardiorespiratory machines. It is recommended that you perform five to ten minutes of easy to moderate yet continuous cardiorespiratory exercise to begin your warm-up.

HOW TO MONITOR YOUR WARM-UP LEVELS

Unless you are wearing a heart rate monitor, there is no way to determine what your exact heart rate is. In this case you can use what trainers refer to as the rate of perceived exertion. This means that you monitor your intensity by how you are feeling. On a scale of 1–20, with 1 being the easiest and 20 being all-out, 100 percent effort, the warm-up should start at a 3 or 4, increase to 5 or 6 after a few minutes, then increase to 7 or 8 after a few more minutes. The warm-up usually does not go over a 10 on the intensity scale.

"Blueberries contain disease-fighting, age-proofing antioxidants and anticancer properties. They help lower cholesterol levels, help prevent short-term memory loss, and help promote weight control."

—Jonny Bowden, PhD, CNS

Make Every Day a Fresh Blueberry Day

In a *Newsweek* article dated June 17, 2002, neuroscientist James Joseph of Tufts University made it clear that when it comes to brain protection, there's nothing quite like the blueberry. Dr. Joseph calls it the "brain berry" and attributes its health benefits to antioxidant and anti-inflammatory compounds. He sees potential for reversing short-term memory loss and forestalling many other effects of aging. The American Institute for Cancer Research recommends eating blueberries because they are "one of the best sources of antioxidants, substances that can slow the aging process and reduce cell damage that can lead to cancer."

By eating only half a cup of fresh or frozen blueberries a day, you can receive their antioxidant protection and benefit from their anti-aging and metabolism-boosting properties. When out of season, use frozen blueberries in a smoothie or mixed with yogurt and walnuts as a delicious snack.

THAT'S BERRY GOOD NEWS!

Eating a diet rich in blackberries, blueberries, raspberries, cranberries, and strawberries may help to reduce your risk of several types of cancer. The blue color in blueberries comes from anthocyanins, phytochemicals that help protect your body from cancer. Blueberries and raspberries also contain lutein, which is important for healthy vision.

"If you're working out in front of a mirror and watching your muscles grow, your ego has reached a point where it is now eating itself. That's why I believe there should be a psychiatrist at every health club, so that when they see you doing this, they will take you away for a little chat."

—Lewis Black

Be Patient and Avoid Overtraining

A major reason that new athletes overtrain is that they don't see progress fast enough. Even veterans can fall into that trap, and the resulting additional stress only adds to the negative energy that hampers training even more.

As you get into your training, it may seem at times that you have stayed at a certain level for a long time. Perhaps your goal is to be able to run a mile in eight minutes, and you just can't seem to cover the distance much faster than nine minutes. Is the solution to run twice as much or do your workouts twice as fast? No, and the likely results of overdoing it have already been covered.

It's normal for your training to progress in plateaus. You may be surprised and a bit chagrined at the time it takes you to go from one level to the next. It is worth noting that athletes can spend years progressing from level to level. Don't be discouraged if you feel that your progress is slower than it should be. Wait for the breakthroughs. They will come.

One way to assure that your training progresses is to get adequate rest. This is especially important after an intense workout. When resting, your body rebuilds muscles that have been broken down by the stresses of training. If you never give your muscles a break, they can't rebuild efficiently. The results can be injury and burnout—or both.

"When the body gets working appropriately, the force of gravity can flow through. Then, spontaneously, the body heals itself."

—Ida Rolf

Get a Sports Massage

One of the best things you can do to improve flexibility in your muscles and tendons is to get a sports massage. Sports massage can alleviate muscle strains and spasms and help flush toxins, primarily lactic acid, from your system. A massage can target a certain area or cover the whole body according to the your needs. A good massage practitioner gets to know each client's body and can focus efforts where they are needed most.

There are two kinds of massage techniques that can be very effective for athletes.

- Traditional sports massage that focuses on the muscles and tendons you use in your sport.
- Structural Integration (SI), sometimes called Rolfing (after the creator of the technique, Ida P. Rolf). The basic SI principle is that misalignment of the muscles and joints can cause a lot of problems. Undergoing SI can be very intense, but many athletes swear by the process and the results of SI therapy.

It could well be worth your while to investigate both disciplines, but it would be a mistake to expect miracles from either, certainly not in one or two sessions. For best results, find a good massage therapist and schedule sessions at least once a month. Your body will thank you for it.

"I have been coaching recently. I coached high school basketball in Arizona, and I hope that more opportunities become available."

—Kareem Abdul-Jabbar

Coach a Children's Sports Team

If you have children, you already know how much they love to run while playing games in the yard or at school. You can help them develop an appreciation for teamwork and good sportsmanship by coaching their team in T-ball, soccer, gymnastics, synchronized swimming, football, track and field, or other sports. Children are naturally happy and enthusiastic. Volunteer to serve as their coach and share in their joy when they play. You may discover that winning or losing really isn't as important as how they play the game.

And, in the meantime, you'll be getting lots of fresh air and exercise. Don't wait, sign up today!

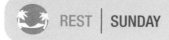
"Dawn: When men of reason go to bed."

—Ambrose Bierce

Chill Out If You Can't Sleep

Don't get all stressed out about not being able to get to sleep. An occasional night of too-few ZZZs won't hurt you as long as you usually get enough sleep. Rather than lying in the dark, tossing and turning in frustration, turn on the light and find something to read. Get comfortable. Sip some warm milk or chamomile tea. Meditate. Steer your mind away from worries and think about pleasant things—not sleep, just pleasant things. Breathe. Even if you don't get to sleep, at least you'll get to relax. And you'll probably feel drowsy soon.

However, if it becomes a pattern that keeps happening, figure out why. Maybe you've been working right up to the time you crawl beneath the sheets, not giving your mind enough time to transition from stress to rest. Perhaps you've been watching the news or a television show that riled up feelings. Once you identify what could be contributing and have tried our suggestions in Week Fourteen, if the problem continues, by all means talk to your doctor about it. Studies show that two thirds of Americans have never been asked by their doctors how well they sleep, but 80 percent have never brought up the subject with their doctors, either. Tell your doctor you are concerned about your sleep problems. He or she may have a simple solution.

"If it weren't for the fact that the TV set and the refrigerator are so far apart, some of us wouldn't get any exercise at all."

—Joey Adams

Make Healthy Snacks Part of Your Eating Plan for the Day

Eating daily snacks is a great way to make sure your metabolism is at its peak—as long as you're choosing healthy foods that provide important nutrients, and not a lot of fat or calories.

A healthy snack should be portion sensitive—a small amount of something nutritious—to keep the metabolic fires burning and tide you over to your next meal. Snacks should be small amounts of nutrient-dense foods ideally consisting of protein and carbohydrate. A few whole-wheat crackers with a wedge of farmer's cheese; a quarter-cup of cottage cheese with half an orange; a hard-boiled egg and half an apple; a slice of whole-wheat toast with thinly spread peanut butter—just enough to provide a steady source of energy throughout the day or to stave off hunger that would cause you to overeat at your next meal.

Here's how to snack smartly:

- Choose whole-grain products: Whole grains are rich in fiber and complex carbohydrates, so they boost your metabolism for longer periods because they require more effort to digest.
- Have a fruit or vegetable: Fruits and vegetables are filled with vitamins, minerals, and fiber. They will fill you up without adding many calories to your diet.
- Nibble on a handful of nuts or seeds: They provide protein and monounsaturated fat, so they help you feel full longer. Just don't eat more than a small handful because they're also high in calories.
- Try low-fat dairy products: Cheese, yogurt, and other dairy products are good sources of calcium, protein, and many other vitamins and minerals, but read the labels to make sure you're not eating added sugars.

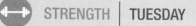
"Whenever you go for a run, your muscles have to contract with more force and at a faster rate than when at rest. The only way your muscles can contract is if they've been provided the necessary oxygen by your blood. No oxygen, no work—it's pretty simple."

—Tina Angelotti, fitness instructor, Krav Maga National Training Center

Increase Your Cardiorespiratory Strength and Endurance

Cardiorespiratory (cardio meaning heart and respiratory meaning lungs) fitness is the ability to utilize large muscle groups for physical activity at a moderate or high intensity or prolonged periods of time. Your cardiorespiratory system—your heart, lungs, blood vessels, circulatory system, and blood—must reach every cell in your body and constantly respond to any changes within your body in order to keep all the organs and systems functioning properly. To build strength and endurance, you need to increase your cardiorespiratory fitness. Here are two treadmill workouts to get you started:

Treadmill Workout 1

1. Start with a brisk walk. For most people this will be at a speed of about 3.5–4 miles per hour.
2. Walk for 2–3 minute intervals. Every 2–3 minutes, increase your pace by .2 mph until you reach a point where you feel as though you are working moderately hard.
3. Maintain this moderately difficult pace for an additional 2 minutes. Decrease your pace by .2 (1/5) mph every 2 minutes after that. Continue to do so until your pace returns to a brisk walk.
4. Repeat this cycle 2–3 times.

Treadmill Workout 2

1. Begin with a brisk walk for 2–3 minutes.
2. When ready, begin a light jog for another 2–3 minutes (5.0–5.5 mph).
3. Increase the incline to 1.0 and continue jogging for 2–3 minutes.
4. Increase the incline to 2.0 and continue for 2–3 minutes.
5. Increase the incline to 3.0 and continue for 2–3 minutes.
6. Bring the incline back to 1.0 and continue for 2–3 minutes.
7. Repeat this cycle 2–3 times.

*"We don't stop playing because we grow old;
we grow old because we stop playing."*

—George Bernard Shaw

Stimulate Your Brain by Playing What's in a Name?

Find words using only the letters in a given name. Each letter in a name can be used only once in your word. For example, if the name is George Washington, then you could make the words *soar, grow, note,* and many others. Words that are always capitalized or require a hyphen or an apostrophe are not included in the answer lists. Words with variant or British spellings are also not included. Try this one:

Liam Neeson

Find 10 five-letter words:

1. _____
2. _____
3. _____
4. _____
5. _____
6. _____
7. _____
8. _____
9. _____
10. _____

aeons, aisle, alien, alims, aloes, aloin, alone, amies, amine, amino, amins, amole, anele, anile, anils, anime, anion, anise, anole, elain, elans, elemi, eloin, enema, enols, eosin, inane, lames, lanes, leans, lease, leman, lemon, lenes, lenis, lenos, lense, liane, leone, liens, liman, limas, limen, limes, limns, linen, lines, lions, loams, loans, loins, lomas, maile, mails, mains, males, manes, manos, manse, mason, meals, means, melon, mensa, mense, mesan, meson, miens, miles, milos, minae, minas, mines, moans, moils, molas, moles, monas, monie, nails, names, neems, nemas, neons, nines, noels, noils, noise, nomas, nomen, nomes, nonas, noles, olein, omens, salmi, salon, seine, semen, senna, slain, slime, smile, elite, solan, solei

snail, solan, solei

"The fatigue produced on the muscles of the human frame does not altogether depend on the actual force employed in each effort, but partly on the frequency with which it is exerted."

—Charles Babbage

Don't Ignore Pain

Only the easiest of workouts will be pain free. The stress of pushing your muscles and tendons to another level, which is how you gain in strength and endurance, will bring some discomfort. For example, if you are doing some hill training, running or biking, it's going to hurt as you push yourself up that incline. If your swim session is focused on increasing your speed, your shoulders will be burning as you get to the end of the pool each time.

All that is normal. It is an entirely different matter when you experience unexpected or sharp pain. When that happens, the alarm bells should start going off. It is a mistake with potentially serious consequences to ignore acute pain or to train through it.

Whatever you are doing, if you feel a sharp pain, stop your activity. Walk if you are running, coast if you are biking, get to the side of the pool (or out of it) if you are swimming. Give yourself a few minutes, then resume whatever you were doing. If the pain persists, it's time to head home.

If sharp pain doesn't go away with a brief break from your activity, and when it comes back even after a couple of days off, you may be dealing with a potentially serious issue. Sometimes rest and ice will do the trick, even extra stretching in some cases. If the recommended treatments don't bring relief, find a physician, preferably one who knows sports injuries, who can more easily diagnose your problem and prescribe the most effective treatments. More important, a sports doctor will also detect the more serious problems that, untreated, can lead to long periods of inactivity.

"It's been told that swimming is a wimp sport, but I don't see it. We don't get timeouts, in the middle of a race we can't stop and catch our breath, we can't roll on our stomachs and lie there, and we can't ask for a substitution."

—Dusty Hicks

Give Your Overworked Muscles a Break, Go for a Swim

For the compulsive athlete, swimming is one of the best cross-training activities to add to your regimen. Swimming gives tired muscles a breather while providing an excellent upper body workout. Additionally, water has a therapeutic effect on all muscle groups.

If you swim for the aerobic benefit, do not be concerned that your heart rate does not get as high as during other activities. The loss of gravitational force, the horizontal position, and the cooling effect of the water temperature all contribute toward keeping your heart rate low.

A low heart rate does not mean that your aerobic efforts are in vain. Remember, aerobic exercise is about oxygen utilization, and the heart rate mirrors what is happening on an oxygen level. But in this case, the mirror gives a distorted picture of what's really going on. Even though swimming conditions yield relatively lower heart rate numbers, your body is still processing oxygen, and that's what counts. A general rule is that the swimming heart rate is typically 10–20 beats per minute less than that for dry land activities.

WHY SWIMMING REJUVENATES YOUR MUSCLES

Swimming is a good buffer for muscle soreness. It is a low-impact activity that you can do with a lower heart rate. Swimming is a great way to flush toxins such as lactic acid from your system the day after an intense running or cycling workout.

"If you have ever raked, hoed, or weeded a garden bed, you already know that gardening is a good workout."

—Jeff Restuccio, author of *Fitness the Dynamic Gardening Way*

Plant a Vegetable Garden and Eat the Produce

You consciously choose to eat healthier, avoid purchasing packaged foods, and buy organic whenever possible. Still, how can you be certain that your food hasn't been treated in some way with agents you want to avoid (such as those that may cause cancer)? Try growing your own food. Plant a postage stamp–sized garden and do companion plantings, (that is, placing plants known to repel specific pests next to plants that attract those pests) to keep down the pest population. You don't need much space for a small kitchen garden, but if space is a major consideration, you can grow your veggies in pots and planters on the patio. Freshly picked tomatoes, peppers, and other vegetables taste far superior and have greater nutritional value than those shipped and warehoused. You'll be both healthier and happier eating organic food from your garden.

HOW TO GET A WORKOUT GARDENING

Regular garden chores can burn anywhere from 120 to 200 calories per half hour, depending on the intensity of the activity. To maximize benefits from gardening, focus on the major muscle groups, bend your knees while raking, or place a crate that requires you to step up and down as you move from one flower bed to the next. It is important to start stretching for several weeks prior to beginning outdoor spring chores. Crunches, leg and arm lifts, squats, and even push ups can help prepare those dormant muscles for spring and summer chores.

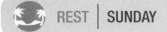

"For sleep, one needs endless depths of blackness to sink into;
daylight is too shallow, it will not cover one."

—Anne Morrow Lindbergh

Create a Bedtime Ritual for Yourself

Parents are often advised to give their sleep-resistant children a routine, but the technique works for grownups, too. Your routine should include a series of steps that are conducive to relaxation—for example, a bath or shower, then perhaps a few minutes of deep breathing or other relaxation technique; a cup of herbal tea; a good book instead of the television or computer; swapping back rubs, neck rubs, or foot rubs with a partner; writing in your journal. Then, it's lights out.

ARE YOU SUFFERING FROM SLEEP DEPRIVATION?

Sleep deprivation has a specific and dramatic physical effect on the body. The average adult requires 8 hours of sleep per night, and teenagers require 8.5 to 9.25 hours. If you don't get enough sleep, you may be experiencing the following:

- Increased irritability
- Depression
- Anxiety
- Decreased ability to concentrate and understand information
- Increased likelihood of making mistakes and having accidents
- Increased clumsiness and slower reaction times (dangerous behind the wheel)
- A suppressed immune system
- Undesirable weight gain

"Soup and fish explain half the emotions of human life."

—Sydney Smith

Make Sure You Get Enough Calcium

Calcium is an important part of a balanced diet because it helps strengthen bones, helps regulate your blood pressure, helps secrete hormones and digestive enzymes, assists directly with weight loss, regulates heart muscle function, and helps boost your metabolism.

The easiest way to stock up on your calcium needs is by eating dairy products like milk, cheese, and yogurt. But there are many other foods that are also rich in calcium. They include dark green leafy vegetables like broccoli, spinach, kale, and collards; fish with edible bones; calcium-fortified soy milk; tofu made with calcium; shelled almonds; turnips; mustard greens; sesame seeds; blackstrap molasses; calcium-fortified cereals; and calcium-fortified orange juice.

"During most sports and recreational activities, your heart rate will reach levels that are very high. Your body should be trained for this kind of physiological demand."

—Jeff Levine, Krav Maga instructor

Use a Stationary Bike to Strengthen Your Cardiorespiratory System

Stationary cycling (or *spinning*, as it's also called) is a popular fitness trend. Widespread availability of stationary bikes makes them excellent supplementary tools for fitness training, particularly when used to slowly strengthen your cardiorespiratory system. Here are two stationary bike routines that will help you improve your heart and lung function:

Stationary Bicycle Workout 1

1. 3 minutes with resistance at 8 (or equivalent for your machine).
2. 1 minute with resistance at 9 (or equivalent for your machine).
3. 1 minute with resistance at 10 (or equivalent).
4. 1 minute with resistance at 9 (or equivalent).
5. 1 minute with resistance at 8 (or equivalent).
6. Repeat this cycle 3–5 times.

Stationary Bicycle Workout 2

1. 3 minutes with resistance at 10 (or equivalent).
2. Keep resistance at 10 (or equivalent) and speed up the legs for 15 seconds.
3. Keep resistance at 10 (or equivalent) and slow down for 15 seconds.
4. Continue alternating your rpms every 15 seconds for a total of 3 minutes.
5. Recover and repeat the cycle at resistance 11 then at 12 (or equivalents).

"You can undergo an emotional reeducation. By meditative exertion and other mental exercises, you can actively change your feelings, your attitudes, and your mind-set."

—Francisca Cho, Buddhist scholar

Meditate to Stimulate Your Brain

For eons, experts believed meditation calmed the brain, and it does, but it also activates the most thoughtful part of your brain. Studies have found that effective meditation increases blood flow to the brain and balances brain wave patterns. It also boosts the immune system and improves cognitive function, including memory. It balances your state of mind, increases creativity, increases sense of peace, increases awareness, bolsters positive thinking, elevates your consciousness, and builds confidence and wisdom. In other words, meditation does a whole lot of good for your brain. There are many kinds of meditation; choose one that works for you.

Here are two online audio resources for meditations:

- Mindfulness Awareness Research Center (MARC) at UCLA offers a selection of audio files you can listen to or download. One provides complete meditation instructions, and others offer a variety of options, time-wise and content-wise. Once you've familiarized yourself with the technique, you can then opt for mindfulness meditations ranging from three minutes to twelve minutes. There are short and long versions of a breathing meditation, a body and sound meditation, and a loving kindness meditation, among others. See *http://marc.ucla.edu*.
- You can also find a wealth of audio CDs and digital downloads on everything from Qigong to Taoist to Kabbalah meditations; Tibetan, Buddhist, Vipassana, and Zen practices; and guided meditations from teachers such as Pema Chödrön, Jack Kornfield, Thich Nhat Hanh, Jon Kabat-Zinn, and many others on *http://soundstrue.com*.

"I was in the gym five days a week, two hours a day. At one point, I was going seven days straight. I had put on a lot of weight, and then I started losing it drastically, so I was worried. It turned out I was overworking myself. My trainer told me that I couldn't break a sweat, because I was burning more calories than I was putting on."

—Taylor Lautner

Take at Least One Day Off a Week

It's human nature to think that if four days of training a week are good, then seven must be ideal. Too bad there isn't an eighth day! Get that notion out of your mind right now, especially if you are new to physical activity. Even top athletes build rest days into their training schedules, and they know why it's important.

Exercise and strength training tear down your muscles. They grow stronger in the process of being rebuilt. That's the wonder of the human body. If you never give your body a chance to rest, the rebuilding process won't occur or it won't be as efficient. Injury is the inevitable result of nonstop training.

Those who are new to sports should have at least one day a week with no exercise at all. If you schedule only one day of complete rest (doing little or nothing), you should avoid hard workouts two days in a row. Any time you have an intense workout, it should be followed the next day with something easy—or even a day off if you do not feel fully recovered.

"The breaking wave and the muscle as it contracts obey the same law. Delicate line gathers the body's total strength in a bold balance. Shall my soul meet so severe a curve, journeying on its way to form?"

—Dag Hammarskjold

Maintain Your Ability to Balance

The body is always looking to find a state of equilibrium. As you age, this process that is controlled by the nervous system begins to slow down. This slowing down process is inevitable, but with training you can prolong the process and live life to the fullest whatever your age.

Practicing balance exercises challenges the nervous system and helps keep the mind-body connection sharp. It also helps to keep the mind and body sharp in the case that balance has to be regained. It has happened to us all at some point—tripping over a parking block or missing that last step. Without any balance practice your response to regaining balance is slow. In the instance that you may be falling, it is crucial to be able to regain balance quickly.

WHY YOU SHOULD START YOUNG TO IMPROVE YOUR BALANCE

Human beings lose most of their natural balance after age twenty-five. This is part of the reason that elderly people can fall so easily. If they do not practice maintaining balance, they can easily lose balance, possibly leading to a fall that could result in a serious injury.

"It becomes increasingly clear through research on the brain as well as in other parts of study, that childhood needs play. Play acts as a forward feed mechanism into courageous, creative, rigorous thinking in adulthood."

—Tina Bruce, Professor, London Metropolitan University

Play Outside with Your Kids

Children need to play, and so do you. Play is a marvelous way to relax and to be physically active. Here are some ideas on activities you can do as a family together:

- Play games like tag or hide-and-seek instead of watching television.
- Do chores like cleaning the garage or the yard, going grocery shopping, or walking the dog. If you make it fun, they'll jump at the chance to spend time with you.
- Shoot hoops in the back yard or go to a neighborhood school or park.
- Go bicycle riding, in-line skating, or hiking.

Not only will the whole family get in shape together, but you'll also enjoy more family time doing group activities.

"Summer is the time when one sheds one's tensions with one's clothes, and the right kind of day is jeweled balm for the battered spirit. A few of those days and you can become drunk with the belief that all's right with the world."

—Ada Louise Huxtable

Lift Your Mood with Sage and Lemon Balm Extract

Professor Elaine Perry, of the University of Newcastle upon Tyne in northern England, told members of a medical conference on the psychiatry of old age held in February 2004 that the plant extracts of sage and lemon balm produced promising results in studies to improve memory and behavior in Alzheimer's patients. Dr. Perry said: "In controlled trials in normal volunteers, both extracts improved memory, and lemon balm improved mood. Lemon balm reduced agitation and improved quality of life in people with Alzheimer's disease."

If you've had a stressful week, burn a lemon or sage scented candle, or slather on a lemon-scented lotion.

"Take all that is given whether wealth, love or language, nothing comes by mistake and with good digestion all can be turned to health."

—George Herbert

Boost Probiotics by Eating Active Culture Yogurt

Yogurt is an excellent source of calcium that also provides about 9 grams of animal protein per 6-ounce serving, plus vitamin B_2, vitamin B_{12}, potassium, and magnesium. One of the most beneficial aspects of yogurt comes from the use of active, good bacteria known as probiotics. Probiotics adjust the natural balance of organisms, known as microflora, in the intestines to aid digestion. To make sure your favorite brand of yogurt contains active cultures, look for labeling that says "live and active cultures," or for words such as *Bifidus regularis*, *L. bulgaricus*, *S. thermophilus*, or *Bifidobacterium*. Here's a tasty and healthy treat using yogurt:

CRUNCHY CREAMY YOGURT PARFAIT

Serves 1
2 tablespoons bran flakes cereal
4 ounces sugar-free vanilla yogurt
¼ cup sliced strawberries

Layer the ingredients in a tall cup, starting with the bran flakes, then the yogurt, and finally the strawberries.

PER SERVING: Calories 210 | **Fat** 1g | **Protein** 9g | **Sodium** 295mg | **Fiber** 6g | **Carbohydrates** 46g

"If a regular schedule of balance training is not maintained, even athletes will begin to find it more difficult to exhibit the high level of grace and stability that is required of them."

—Nathan Brown, martial arts instructor

Improve Your Static Balance by Doing a Single-Leg Standing Pose

Balance is the ability to maintain equilibrium against the force of gravity. It is a basic skill needed in everyday life. Although the inner ear is the balance center, in order to balance, you need strong muscles and joints. There are two types of balance: static and dynamic.

Static balance is exactly what it sounds like—holding a position and not moving. Standing on one leg and holding the other knee up (stork stand) is a static balance exercise. Begin the single-leg standing pose with the knee of one of your legs lifted up in front of you. Your opposite leg, which is going to be your standing/support leg, should be completely straight. Next, take your bent leg and extend it out in front of you as straight and as high as you can. If your standing leg is bending in order to balance you, then you are not ready to hold your leg so high and you will need to lower your extended leg a bit for the moment. As you improve and become more stable in this pose you will be able to lift the extended leg higher. Avoid lifting your extended leg beyond the point where you can maintain balance while keeping both of your legs straight. Bending your knees is compensating for a lack of strength or flexibility, so it's more important for you to maintain the alignment than to lift your leg as high as possible. Don't forget to alternate legs!

"Fitness: If it came in a bottle, everybody would have a great body."

—Cher

Challenge Your Nervous System by Tossing a Ball Around

For many years teachers and pediatricians assumed that the correct development of movement was important to the development of intelligence in children because it challenged students mentally as well as physically. The motor skills involved in sending different left and right combinations with your hands or legs require the nervous system to recall or remember how to do these complex movements in the correct order. Many undergoing Krav Maga fitness training, in particular, have reported an increase in memory. Other people have reported being able to think faster on their feet as a result of fitness training.

Movements or exercises that challenge any skill-related components of fitness—such as balance, agility, coordination, speed, power, or reaction time—enhance one's cognitive functioning. For example, hand-eye coordination exercises, such as tossing a medicine ball back and forth, may seem simple, but they can provide a challenge that is good for your mental agility.

Try tossing the ball while balancing on one foot. If that still feels simple, have your partner toss the ball at different angles. Incrementally changing a simple exercise challenges the nervous system and keeps individuals concentrating and focused on their performance. Every time you challenge the nervous system, you are training the brain to think more efficiently.

"Most of the time I meet my trainer at the gym and we do a lot of everything: weights circuit with cardio, football drills, sprinting with weights on the treadmill."

—Charisma Carpenter

Try a Split Routine

As with many things in life, when it comes to weight training, more is not necessarily better. Muscles need at least forty-eight hours in between training sessions to recover and repair. (The one exception is the abdominal muscle group, which can be exercised every day.) If you're training your entire body daily, your muscles will not have time to build new tissue. You could be overtraining. Many advanced bodybuilders divide their body parts into two groups and exercise them alternately on consecutive days. This is known as working a "split routine."

For example, work your upper body by lifting weights one day, and then the next day focus on squats or other legwork. You could also spend one day on the elliptical trainer, and the next day working on your upper body strength. Running one day and swimming the next day would also be an effective way to give stressed muscles the needed time to recuperate. Swimming, in general, is an excellent interim activity.

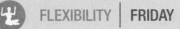

"People have been practicing yoga for thousands of years because they get something out of it."

—Cynthia Worby, MSW, MPH, RYT

No More Yoga Excuses! Sign Up for a Class Today!

Everyone can do yoga regardless of age, size, flexibility, or health. Many people unfamiliar with yoga think that they have to be like a Gumby toy—able to touch their toes to their nose—but this is not true. Yoga is the great equalizer. Two people can walk into a yoga class, one very flexible with no strength and the other stiff (too strong) with little flexibility. The same poses done by these individuals will tighten up the overly flexible person and loosen the stiff person. Overweight people, pregnant women, and older people can practice yoga and receive its benefits. There are many types of yoga suitable for anyone and poses can *always* be modified to fit an individual's needs. Search online for yoga studios near you, and then call several to find the one that feels most right. If you have specific concerns, talk them over with the yoga instructor prior to your first class.

YOGA AS A PAIN RELIEVER

Yoga is a marvelous therapeutic tool. Many ailments and disorders can be relieved by specific postures and breathing practices under the guidance of a qualified yoga teacher. Often, people are amazed to find their backaches, headaches, and joint pain can disappear with regular practice. People with cancer, cardiac problems, and multiple sclerosis can experience relief of some symptoms and develop the ability to relax more fully and cope with stress.

"Base Ball, to be played thoroughly, requires the possession of muscular strength, great agility, quickness of eye, readiness of hand, and many other faculties of mind and body that mark the man of nerve."

—Henry Chadwick

Join a Softball League

Getting active and staying active provides exercise and uplifts your mood. If you prefer team sports to those you do solo, join a softball team or organize one that includes people from your circle of friends or business colleagues. Softball teams play other players, so even as you are having fun with friends on your team you are also potentially making new friends with players from other teams. Psychologists say those who live isolated lives or without strong social networks are not as happy as those who have strong bonds, social connections, and ongoing support from friends and family.

By signing up for a league, you'll also be responsible for showing up for league play every week and expected to do your best. That pressure might inspire you to the batting cages during the week to practice in anticipation of the upcoming game. Invite your friends out to watch you play if you need a little more incentive to play well. As you strive to get a home run or increase your strike potential, you'll probably start working out a little more often on the side.

If you've had a hard time staying committed to exercising, joining one of these leagues means you'll be burning 365 extra calories an hour, at least one day a week. That, hopefully, will help convince you that burning calories doesn't have to be a chore and can involve bonding, friendship, and even laughter!

"The revival interest in herbal medicine is a worldwide phenomenon."
—Mark Blumenthal, Executive Director of the American Botanical Council

Calm Yourself with Herbal Remedies

If you are feeling particularly anxious, herbal remedies have often proved helpful. Here are two that many have found effective:

Try Valerian Instead of Valium

Called "the Valium of the nineteenth century" (though it has no chemical similarity to Valium), the herb valerian (*Valeriana officinalis*) is a common sedative used worldwide. In Europe, it is prescribed for anxiety. Herbalists have chosen valerian for treatment of nervous tension and even for panic attacks. It is known as a safe non-narcotic herbal sedative and is often combined with other herbs to make pain-relieving remedies, as it has the ability to relax muscle spasms. Despite the fact that valerian has been widely studied, just how it works remains a mystery.

Try Snakeroot

For centuries, the plant Indian snakeroot was used in Ayurvedic medicine for a range of problems, including anxiety, headache, fevers, and snakebites. Mahatma Gandhi was reputed to drink a cup of snakeroot tea at bedtime if he had had a busy day and felt overstimulated. Western herbalists valued it as a powerful tranquilizer and also used it to treat high blood pressure.

Then, in 1947, scientists at the CIBA company extracted the alkaloid reserpine from snakeroot and began marketing a drug called Serpasil for high blood pressure. This drug proved to have many unpleasant side effects, and in the 1950s, a new tranquilizer was developed from the herb. This has always been a prescription-only drug in the United States, but in other parts of the world, including Europe and Asia, snakeroot in its natural state continues to be widely used as a soothing tea and tranquilizer.

"Happiness lies, first of all, in health."

—George William Curtis

Blend a Power-Packed Vitamin C Smoothie

Not only is vitamin C a strong vitamin most well known for illness prevention, it works absolute wonders in many areas of promoting optimal health. In addition to being a strong supporter of bone health by improving the collagen-building process, building and retaining quality muscle, and improving the efficiency of blood vessels, it actually aids in the body's absorption of iron. Common mineral deficiencies can be reversed by including an abundance of vitamin C with your daily intake of iron-rich foods. Here's a vitamin C–packed smoothie recipe, intensified by the addition of ginger, vitamin K, and iron-rich spinach.

VITAMIN C CANCER PREVENTION

Recipe Yields: 3–4 cups

1 cup spinach
1 grapefruit, peeled
1 cup pineapple, peeled and cored
1 orange, peeled
a small slice of whole ginger, peeled
1 cup purified water

1. Combine spinach, grapefruit, pineapple, orange, ginger, and ½ cup water in a blender and blend until thoroughly combined.
2. Add remaining ½ cup water as needed while blending until desired consistency is achieved.

PER 1 CUP SERVING: Calories 62 | **Fat** 0g | **Protein** 1g | **Sodium** 8mg | **Fiber** 2g | **Carbohydrates** 16g

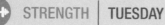

"I have two doctors, my left leg and my right."

—G. M. Trevelyan

Improve Your Dynamic Balance by Practicing Kicks

Dynamic balance dictates your ability to maintain a level equilibrium while you are in motion. Most martial arts are quite dependent upon dynamic balance. A spin kick, such as you would often see in tae kwon do, can very easily throw the deliverer off balance if that person has not practiced the maneuver enough to maintain balance during its execution. Dynamic balance requires your center of mass (COM) to stay over your base of support to maintain balance in any movement. Your COM is generally located just below your navel and in an inch. The base of support is whatever part of your body is touching the ground. That may be your feet, your hands, or, if you are working on movement on the ground, the side of your body. Your center of mass needs to stay over your base of support to maintain balance in any movement.

Single-leg repetition kicks are a great way to strengthen your dynamic balance. Begin by standing on your left leg, as you bring your right knee forward and up. As your hips move forward, extend your right foot out to complete the kick. Send it out and back in repetition, touching the ball of your foot back on the floor lightly between each kick. Remember, your target is the groin or midsection of an imagined opponent.

This can also be done with a round kick. Turn the base foot out, lift the kicking leg knee up, and extend the kick out and back and again lightly touch the foot to the floor between each kick. Be sure you recoil the kick as this will help you stay balanced. The target for a round kick would be someone's rib cage. When performing exercises that train dynamic balance, you should perform eight to twelve repetitions and anywhere from one to three sets.

"The nice thing about doing a crossword puzzle is, you know there is a solution."

—Stephen Sondheim

Challenge Your Brain by Playing Scrambled Categories

Unscramble the letters to form words. All of the words in each group belong in the given category. You will be able to unscramble some of these immediately, while others will take more thought.

Parts of a Book

1. INSEP _____
2. GPSEA _____
3. OVCRE _____
4. KECATJ _____
5. BGIDINN _____

What Does Your Garden Grow?

1. CNOR _____
2. UHAQSS _____
3. AEOMOTTS _____
4. ROSTCRA _____
5. EWTNMOLAER _____

Sports

1. BAELAKLTSB _____
2. SLALEBAB _____
3. LFOLOBTA _____
4. KCHEYO _____
5. COECSR _____

ANSWERS:

Parts of a Book
1. Spine
2. Pages
3. Cover
4. Jacket
5. Binding

What Does Your Garden Grow?
1. Corn
2. Squash
3. Tomatoes
4. Carrots
5. Watermelon

Sports
1. Basketball
2. Baseball
3. Football
4. Hockey
5. Soccer

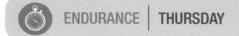

"Ability is what you are capable of doing. Motivation determines what you do. Attitude determines how well you do it."

—Lou Holtz

Stay Motivated to Stick with Your Training Program

Many people find it easier to start rather than stick with a training program. Fifty percent of people drop out of training programs within six months. Once you get past the six-month mark, it is likely that it has become part of your lifestyle and continuing it won't be a problem. The following is a list of Training Continuation Tips that people who exercise as part of their daily lives use to keep themselves motivated.

- Tailor the intensity, duration, and frequency of training sessions to your level.
- Exercise with a friend.
- Find or make a convenient place to exercise.
- Utilize music that motivates you.
- Set realistic goals.
- Keep an exercise journal.
- Tell others what you are doing.
- Post notes around your living quarters to remind you of your goals.
- Reward yourself for achieving your goals (but not with pizza and ice cream!) with healthy rewards, such as treating yourself to a relaxing afternoon at a spa or a night at the movies with friends.

"Warrior pose battles inner weakness and wins focus. You see that there is no war within you. You're on your own side, and you are your own strength."

—Terri Guillemets

Learn the Benefits of Yoga Asanas

Asanas are the various geometric postures of yoga. In any pose, there must be a clear action, sense of direction, and center of gravity. In order to maintain the center of gravity the muscles must be properly aligned. Stability of the pelvic and shoulder girdles is essential to the balance and symmetry of the spine. In standing poses, the feet root down, allowing the legs and the spine to lengthen and extend away from the feet. The buttock bones are the foundation in seated poses from which the spine lifts and elongates. In inverted postures, the head, hands, or forearms provide the foundation and stability from which the torso and legs lengthen. The asanas create different effects:

- Standing poses enhance vitality
- Seated poses are calming
- Twists are cleansing
- Supine poses are restful
- Prone poses are energizing
- Inverted postures increase mental strength
- Balancing poses create lightness
- Backbends are exhilarating
- Jumping develops agility

In every pose, for every action there is an equal opposing reaction. Moving in one direction won't create positive change in the body. There cannot be extension without foundation. In every pose, there is a foundation from which extension is possible. This foundation creates the stability and space in the joints, the lengthening of muscle, and the suppleness and correct placement of the organs.

"Farm Aid celebrates the independent family farmers and ranchers who make this country strong, and we know we can only fix the challenges our country faces with the know-how of family farmers."

—Willie Nelson

Frequent Your Local Farmer's Market

Make Saturday the day you visit local farmer's markets. It's not only fun, it's a great way for you to eat fresh foods and support local and family farms, many of which are quickly becoming a thing of the past. Here are other ways you can support local farmers:

- Donate to Farm Aid (*www.farmaid.org*).
- Buy fresh eggs from a local farm. This will help both the farm and you. Your purchase will help with the daily maintenance and possible expansion of the farm. And the fresh eggs will taste better in your omelets, salads, and cakes.
- Buy organic. It costs a little more, but the produce is pesticide free. Animals are treated humanely and animal products and produce often come from smaller farms. You will be supporting local agribusiness committed to taking care of the environment and the people who live in it.

"I put a drop of lavender essential oil on my pillow before I go to sleep."

—Melissa Joan Hart

Experiment with Essential Oils

Today, people all over the world are paying attention to the healing effects of essential oils, and scientists are continuing to conduct research in an attempt to understand more about the effects of these amazing aromas on the human mind, body, and psychology. Essential oils are extracted from the aromatic essences of certain plants, trees, fruits, flowers, herbs, and spices. The collective qualities of each give it a dominant characteristic, whether it be stimulating, calming, energizing, or relaxing. Within the body, essential oils are able to operate in three ways: pharmacologically, physiologically, and psychologically. From the pharmacological perspective, the oils react with body chemistry similarly to drugs, but with a slower and more sympathetic effect and with fewer side effects. The psychological effect is triggered by the connection the aromatic molecules make with the brain.

There are a large number of relaxing aromatic oils on the market, but the best include lavender, sage, sandalwood, frankincense, and chamomile. Some people light scented candles as they relax after a hard day's work or place fragrant potpourri throughout their home. Others prefer to place a few drops of scented oils in their water while they relax in a hot bath or a few drops of scented oil on their pillow to help them unwind and fall asleep faster at night. The important thing is to select a fragrance that is both appealing and relaxing. You may have to experiment until you find the scent that is right for you, but it's well worth the effort. One good Internet source is *Aromaweb.com.*

"Good apple pies are a considerable part of our domestic happiness."

—Jane Austen

Eat More Apples

Apples are fabulous for you—and your metabolism. The active ingredient in apple pulp is pectin, a soluble form of fiber that helps reduce "bad" cholesterol by keeping it in the intestinal tract until it is eliminated. Pectin also creates a sensation of fullness and suppresses appetite. A study published in the *Journal of the National Cancer Institute* shows that pectin binds certain cancer-causing compounds in the colon, accelerating their removal from the body. European studies indicate that apple pectin can even help eliminate lead, mercury, and other toxic heavy metals from the human body. Note: It's important to wash apples thoroughly and to avoid eating the seeds, which can be poisonous. All apples provide super nutrients, but eating different varieties of apples is even better. Here's a delicious recipe for you to try:

OLD-FASHIONED BAKED APPLES

Serves 4
4 baking apples (Romes or Cortlands are good)
8 whole cloves
2 ounces butter (½ stick)
⅓ cup light brown sugar
½ teaspoon ground cinnamon

1. Wash and dry apples thoroughly. Using a small knife, cut a divot from the top of the apples, leaving the stem intact. This "cover" will be replaced when baking. Scoop out the seeds and core with a melon-baller or small spoon. Drop 2 cloves into each apple.
2. Knead together the butter and brown sugar, along with the cinnamon, until it is a paste. Divide equally over the scooped apples, leaving enough space to replace the tops.
3. Place apples in a baking dish, with ½ cup of water on the bottom. Bake at 350 degrees for 1 hour. Sprinkle with cinnamon or powdered sugar before serving.

> *"For those beginning a strength-training program in which the goal is to put on a large amount of muscle tissue, experts may recommend up to 1.7–2 grams of protein per kilogram of body weight—up to two and a half times the recommended amount."*
>
> —Tina Angelotti, developer of the Krav Maga fitness program

Eat More Protein to Help You Build Strong Muscles

Proteins are the main structural material in your body and play a major part of the development of bone, muscle, and other tissues in the body. Although proteins supply some energy, they primarily make your body stronger. Most of your protein likely comes from animal sources such as meat, poultry, and fish, or dairy products, which also carry a significant amount of carbohydrates. Unfortunately, animal proteins have high amounts of cholesterol and saturated fats, which can cause plaque to build up on the walls of blood vessels in your body. Plant-based proteins do not contain cholesterol or saturated fats, unless they are added during food processing. Therefore, animal-based proteins should be consumed with a level of moderation, and your strength-training diet should also include plant-based proteins.

Keep in mind that your body can only process a certain amount of protein for muscular growth. Any proteins above that amount will be used for energy needs or stored as fat or sugar.

Healthy Sources of Dietary Protein

- Lean beef
- Poultry
- Fish
- Legumes
- Broccoli
- Low-fat cottage cheese
- Low-fat yogurt
- Eggs

"If life is just a bowl of cherries, then what am I doing in the pits?"

—Erma Bombeck

Perk Up Your Brain with a Power-Packed Smoothie

Packed with an assortment of vitamins and minerals, an obvious sign from their intense red color, cherries help mental functions like memory. Cherries also improve mental clarity and promote focus and attention. Fire up your brain with this smoothie:

THE SLUMP BUMPER

Recipe Yields: 3–4 cups
1 cup spinach
2 pears, cored and peeled
1 cup cherries, pitted
1 banana, peeled
2 cups almond milk

1. Combine spinach, pears, cherries, banana, and 1 cup of almond milk in a blender and blend until thoroughly combined.
2. Add remaining cup of almond milk while blending until desired texture is achieved.

PER 1 CUP SERVING: Calories 149 | **Fat** 2g | **Protein** 2g | **Sodium** 82mg | **Fiber** 5g | **Carbohydrates** 35g

"It's really unfair to working women in America who read celebrity news and think, 'Why can't I lose weight when I've had a baby?' Well, everyone you're reading about has money for a trainer and a chef. That doesn't make it realistic."

—Rachael Zoe

Hire a Personal Trainer

A personal trainer (PT) is a pro who trains all types of people, from aspiring athletes to fifty-year-old grandmothers. Some specialize while others are jacks of all sports, so to speak. What they all have in common, or should have, is the ability to tailor a fitness or training regimen specifically to the individual being trained. A good personal trainer will first assess your fitness level and test you to see where your weak spots are. The PT will then design a training program to correct any deficiencies and prepare you for your specific goal.

Most personal trainers are athletes, so it is likely your PT will know what you need to achieve what you want in at least a couple of the triathlon sports. If you are really lucky, your trainer will be a triathlete. The benefits of having a personal trainer include the one-on-one attention and instant feedback as you learn proper techniques for your sports. Your PT will be able to assess your limits and design a program that keeps you from overtraining. Most PTs will design workouts with some variety to keep you from being bored with your training while you work the same muscles with different workouts.

Finally, a personal trainer can be your motivator. The PT will take pride in your progress and will naturally want to cheer you on. After all, your success reflects well on your personal trainer.

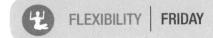

"The beauty is that people often come here for the stretch,
and leave with a lot more."

—Liza Ciano, Yogavermont.com

Ready Yourself for Yoga with Warm-Up Poses

Warm-up poses provide a safe transition into asana practice, isolating muscle groups and body parts, such as the shoulders, the spine, the hips, the lower back, and the groin. You can start with these three warm-up poses this week and add more next week.

- Reclining Mountain Pose: Lie down on your back with your feet together. Stretch your heels and the balls of your feet forward, as you fully stretch your legs away from your feet and ankles. Have your arms diagonally by your sides with the palms facing up.
- Reclining Child's Pose: Lie down on your back with the knees bent and feet flat on the floor. Inhale fully. Exhale and draw the knees into the chest. Hug the knees with the arms and stay for several breaths, savoring the stretching of the lower back muscles. Next, draw your chin toward your knees, and hold for a few breaths.
- The Modified Reclining Child's Pose: Also known as the reclining-hand-on-the-big-toe pose. Still lying down, with your knees bent, extend your left leg onto the floor and stretch the foot forward. Clasp your hands behind your right knee, and hold for several breaths. Then extend your right leg up, either holding behind the knee or holding onto a belt that is around the ball of the right foot. Be in the pose, breathing smoothly, gently stretching the leg or keeping it slightly bent.
- Reclining Child's Pose with Wide Legs: Lying on your back, bend your knees into your chest and then bring your knees comfortably wide apart. Clasp your hands under the knees, holding onto the outside of the knee. Stay in this position for several breaths. Then change the hand position, with the hands on the inside of the knee.

"You have to stay in shape. My grandmother, she started walking five miles a day when she was 60. She's 97 today and we don't know where the hell she is."

—Ellen DeGeneres

Take a Daily Stroll

One of the best forms of exercise that provides a healthful challenge for the human body is walking. It is economical, easy to fit into your day, bears a low risk of injury, and is effective in improving health. Numerous studies show that people who walk regularly have less risk of death or disability from disease.

Studies have shown that people who participate in regular walking programs have higher levels of HDL cholesterol, lower levels of total and LDL cholesterol, and lower levels of triglycerides or blood fats. In addition to reducing these risks of heart disease, walking helps you to enjoy many other benefits, including maintaining a healthy weight, improving the condition of bones and muscles, and reducing stress and tension.

Plus, walking is great. It's easy, fun, and can get you out in the fresh air or can provide an opportunity for socializing with friends while you all shape up together. Walk at a brisk pace for thirty to sixty minutes at least three times each week, and preferably five to six times per week.

TAKE THREE SHORTS WALKS

Short walks contribute to overall health, but they do not constitute fitness workouts. However, short walks are a great addition to an exercise program for mood elevation and for keeping your metabolism rolling along throughout the day. For example, try taking short walks to split up your workday. Take a quick 10-minute walk in the midmorning, a 15-minute walk at lunchtime, and another 10-minute walk in the midafternoon. You'll get a burst of energy, and will probably notice an increase in your productivity.

"The best things in life are nearest: Breath in your nostrils, light in your eyes, flowers at your feet, duties at your hand, the path of right just before you. Then do not grasp at the stars, but do life's plain, common work as it comes, certain that daily duties and daily bread are the sweetest things in life."

—Robert Louis Stevenson

Mindlessly Meditate to Relax

Here is a "mindless" meditation devised to put you into a state of mind that can lead to real rest. To do this meditation—which is really not a meditation at all in any formal sense—recline or lie down comfortably when you can be alone and uninterrupted for an hour. Turn lights down or off and eliminate outside noises and distractions. Close your eyes and let yourself experience the silence around you, then move inward and find a place of silence inside. Let yourself stay in this place as long as you feel comfortable. Begin to follow your breath without trying to alter it. Just feel the quiet rhythm of your SELF. As you do this, let your mind wander wherever it wants to go, like a puppy let outside for an airing. Follow it if you wish, see what interests it, but make no judgments. Think of your mind as a butterfly lighting on one flower, now on another, gathering nectar. Don't push or move your mind in any particular direction. Let it go where it wants. That is the key here. So much meditation tries to harness the mind, tether it like a goat on a rope as bait for large game. Don't do that. As your mind is given the freedom to roam here and there, to play at will, it will lead you to your place of rest.

"Let me pose you a question. Can farm-raised salmon be organic when its feed has nothing to do with its natural diet, even if the feed itself is supposedly organic, and the fish themselves are packed tightly in pens, swimming in their own filth?"

—Mark Bittman

Eat More Wild Salmon

The omega-3 fatty acids present in salmon puts this fish at the top of the superfoods chart. Salmon provides two types of omega-3s: DHA (docosahexaenoic acid) and EPA (eicosapentaenoic acid); and it's high in vitamin D, selenium, protein, and B vitamins. Some studies have found that omega-3s can significantly decrease serum triglyceride levels, lower blood pressure, and reduce blood levels of homocysteine, high levels of which are associated with an increased risk of heart disease, stroke, Alzheimer's disease, Parkinson's disease, and osteoporosis. Omega-3s also help to thin the blood by discouraging platelets in the blood from clumping together, thus reducing the risk that the blood will clot and cause a heart attack. Preliminary research also suggests that omega-3 fatty acids from fish oil may help regulate the rhythm of the heart, as both EPA and DHA have been reported to help prevent cardiac arrhythmias. Potent anti-inflammatory agents, omega-3s help curb an overactive immune system and thus are helpful in the treatment of autoimmune diseases such as rheumatoid arthritis, chronic inflammatory bowel disease, Crohn's disease, and psoriasis. Wild salmon has more nutrients and fewer pollutants than farm-raised salmon so opt for it as often as possible.

WEEK TWENTY-SIX

"The Mayo Clinic cites a number of benefits from core training, which includes strengthening your abs. Among the listed benefits you'll find improved balance, stability and ease of movement plus a toned, attractive midsection and a jump-start toward meeting your fitness goals."

—The Lance Armstrong Foundation

Strengthen Your Abdominal Muscles by Doing Crunches

One of the best, most low-tech ways to strengthen your abdominal muscles is by making abdominal crunches part of your daily workout routine. Here's how to do them:

Lie on your back with your knees bent and feet flat on the floor, about shoulder-width part. Bring your arms up and put your hands under your head, thumbs pointing toward your ears. Don't interlock your fingers, even if your fingers overlap. Keep your head extended from your body so that your chin isn't digging into your chest. Start raising your trunk, curling up from your spine, using your abs—not your hands—to pull yourself up.

Keep your elbows to the side and raise yourself up only enough to lift your shoulder blades off the floor. Pause, then bring your trunk back into position slowly for one repetition. Start by doing 3 sets of 15 reps, adjusting according to whether it feels like too much or not enough.

To increase the intensity of your abdominal crunch workout, try doing your reps with your legs off the floor, crossed at your ankles. Keep your knees bent and your butt on the floor.

"Men do not quit playing because they grow old;
they grow old because they quit playing."

—Oliver Wendell Holmes

Have Fun with Triplet Puzzles

Determine the common word that can be combined with each of the three given words. For example, consider these three words: *trap, prize,* and *out.* The common word is *door,* which makes the answers *trapdoor, door prize,* and *outdoor.* Compounds can be open (*high school*), closed (*schoolhouse*), or hyphenated (*school-age*).

Triplet 1
1. white
2. winner
3. stick

Triplet 3
1. back
2. first
3. held

Triplet 2
1. bed
2. Christmas
3. keeper

Triplet 4
1. bottom
2. blue
3. dumb

"My doctor says I have the body of a 50-year-old."

—Jane Fonda

Beef Up Your Antioxidants

Physical exertion produces free radicals, the bad molecules that can damage tissue and increase inflammation, the body's natural reaction to injury. The damage caused by the free radicals is known as oxidation. Any substance that combats this process is known as an antioxidant. There are a variety of antioxidant supplements you can take, particularly vitamins A, C, E, and B, and there are many fruits that contain antioxidant properties, blueberries being one of the stars in this area.

Another way to combat inflammation is through proteolytic enzyme supplementation. Your body produces these enzymes naturally, but production slows down as you age. Some of the food you eat—cooked or processed meat, for example—causes the enzymes to be diverted from their main role of regulating protein function in the body. Instead, they are used to help the body digest the food. Proteolytic enzymes work against inflammation by neutralizing biochemicals associated with the problem. Between the body's natural slow-down of enzyme production and the diversion of the enzymes for food digestion, you are losing a soldier, so to speak, in the battle against inflammation caused by free radical damage. Supplements work well in replacing those lost enzymes. You can find proteolytic enzyme supplements at any health food store.

Even better is to plan your daily meals to include plenty of fruits and vegetables, which naturally provide the vitamins and minerals you need. Eat healthy so you can play hard and train hard.

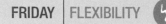
"A photographer gets people to pose for him. A yoga instructor gets people to pose for themselves."

—Terri Guillemets

Add New Yoga Warm-Up Poses

Here are more warm-up poses that provide a safe transition into asana practice, isolating muscle groups and body parts, such as the shoulders, spine, hips, lower back, and groin.

- Supine Spinal Rock: Lying down, with hands clasped under your knees, tuck your chin into your chest and begin rolling up and down your spine, in a gentle, rocking motion. Repeat several times.
- Leg Cradle: Lie down with your knees bent and feet flat on the floor. Bend your right leg out to the side and place the outside of your right ankle on the thigh close to the knee. Clasp your hands under your left knee by threading your right arm between your legs and wrapping your left arm around the outside of your left thigh to the knee. Inhale and, on the exhalation, gently draw your left leg in toward your chest. As you do this, pull your buttocks bones down toward the floor and press your left thigh into your clasped hands. Stay for several breaths and then change sides.
- Stomach-Revolving Pose: Lie down and bend your knees with your feet flat on the floor. Lift your feet away from the floor and bring your knees to your chest. Extend your arms horizontally on the floor. Stack your knees and ankles and let your knees come down to the floor on your right side at a 90-degree angle. Gaze up at the ceiling. Feel your belly and your ribs spiral toward the left. Maintain the length of the spine upon inhalation, twist on the exhalation, and roll your left shoulder down toward the floor (without forcing). Stay in the pose for several breaths, deepening the twist. Then bring your knees back to center and go to the other side.

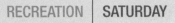
"I travel not to go anywhere, but to go.
I travel for travel's sake. The great affair is to move."

—Robert Louis Stevenson

Make Fitness Your Destination

Take an active vacation, with no goal other than to enjoy yourself and have fun. There are spas with a fitness focus, resorts with activities (skiing, swimming, and skating), walking vacations, biking trips, hiking treks, and far more adventurous options, such as mountain climbing, backwoods cross-country snowshoeing, kayaking, trips during which you learn to sail, and other skill-focused adventures. Whatever your choice, be sure to bring the equipment requested and the right shoes so that you'll be comfortable and able to take part in all the activities.

When you plan your next vacation, consider centering it around physical activity. Build hiking or kayaking or even mountain climbing into your plans or look for an organized event you can participate in. Here are some planned events that offer the opportunity to visit new places, be active in the great outdoors, and meet new people while having fun.

- Bay to Breakers, San Francisco, California
- Bike Ride Around Lake Tahoe, Lake Tahoe, California
- Gasparilla Distance Classic, Tampa, Florida
- Peachtree Road Race, Atlanta, Georgia
- Run to the Far Side, San Francisco, California

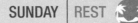
"Just as your car runs more smoothly and requires less energy to go faster and farther when the wheels are in perfect alignment, you perform better when your thoughts, feelings, emotions, goals, and values are in balance."

—Brian Tracy

Make a Ten-Point List of What's Really Important to You

Millions of people live their lives without a sense of direction. Unless you know what is really important to you and what you want out of life, how are you going to know where you are going, how to get what you want, and what your life purpose is? Think of ten things that are really important to you, for example, family unity. Then make each item as specific as possible. Instead of family unity, maybe you really mean eating meals together, working on the chores together, or praying together. Refine the ten things on your list until you know exactly what is of primary importance to you. These are the things that will make you happiest. Knowing what they are can help you make better choices in your personal life journey.

> **EXPRESS GRATITUDE**
>
> Focus on what you love about your life and your emotional brain fires up. You are more coordinated. Write out five things you're grateful for today. Focus on what is making you feel lucky and good about your life. This trains your brain to focus on the love and pleasant experiences in your life. Do it long enough and you'll effectively create a positive groove in your brain.

*"The avocado is a food without rival among
the fruits, the veritable fruit of paradise."*

—David Fairchild

Eat Avocados

Avocados are incredibly healthful for you. In addition to being packed with important vitamins, avocados are able to lower bad cholesterol, decrease your risk for cancer, and prevent heart disease because they include oleic acid (a monounsaturated fat) and healthy fatty acids, and they are high in magnesium and potassium. Research has also shown that these tasty fruits help the body absorb nutrients from other foods eaten with them. Just keep in mind that an avocado is high in calories—each fruit contains approximately 300 calories and 35 grams of fat. Here's one particularly nutritious, low-calorie suggestion:

MEXICAN OMELET FOR ONE

To make this a more muscular Mexican omelet, add 2 tablespoons of black beans for added protein.

¼ cup **Egg Beaters**
Salt and pepper to taste
2 tablespoons salsa
1 slice fat-free Cheddar cheese
½ **sliced avocado**

1. Coat a skillet with nonstick spray. Add Egg Beaters to skillet and salt and pepper to taste. Cook on medium high for 3 minutes.
2. Flip eggs and add salsa and cheese to the center of the eggs. Fold omelet over and cook for another 2 minutes, then flip and cook for an additional 2 minutes. Serve with ½ of a sliced avocado.

PER SERVING (WITHOUT AVOCADO): Calories 225 | **Fat** 17g | **Carbohydrates** 4g | **Protein** 14g | **Sodium** 428mg | **Fiber** 1g

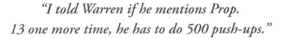
*"I told Warren if he mentions Prop.
13 one more time, he has to do 500 push-ups."*

—Arnold Schwarzenegger

Do Some Good Old-Fashioned Pushups

Pushups are a great way to strengthen your pectoralis major, anterior deltoid, and triceps (chest, shoulder, arms). Kneel on all fours on the floor. Walk your hands forward until your hands are slightly wider than shoulder width apart and your torso resembles a slanted board. Engage your abdominal muscles. Maintain neutral alignment. Straighten your arms and push your body up through your palms. Keep your shoulders relaxed. Maintain neutral alignment.

Inhale to prepare, exhale as you push up. Inhale, return to start. Place a towel under your palms to elevate palms and reduce pressure on your wrists. Another option to reduce pressure on your wrists is to hold onto dumbbells that rest on the floor. Avoid dropping your head. Your pushup should not resemble a nose dive. Avoid locking your elbows when you lift. Lower as low as possible.

If that's a tad too hard, try standing in front of a wall. Place your hands on the wall slightly wider than shoulder width apart. Bend elbows and lower body toward the wall. Straighten arms as you push through hands.

Another option is to kneel on all fours. Lower your chest toward the floor by bending your elbows. Adjust the amount of load by shifting more or less weight from your knees into your hands.

Work your way up to a full body pushup. On floor, instead of working from a slanting board position, extend your legs long and rest on the balls of your feet, so your body resembles a plank.

Add resistance. Assume same body position. Place one end of a rubber exercise band (used to create resistance) under each of your hands and around your back. Push up against the increased resistance of the rubber exercise band. Lower with control.

"It's important to make being active a part of your life, not a segregated activity that requires a big change of routine."

—Jack Raglin, PhD, Kinesiology

Stay Mentally and Physically Active to Maintain Mental Acuity

In 2005, Ohio State University researchers reported that older people who exercised regularly were more likely to maintain the mental acuity they needed to do everyday tasks like follow a recipe and keep track of the pills they take. Some of the recommended mental activities for older people included crossword puzzles, trivia games, Scrabble, card games, and projects, such as fixing appliances and cooking.

A study published in the *Proceedings of the National Academy of Science* (PNAS) in 2001 investigated the benefits of keeping active both mentally and physically during leisure time to prevent Alzheimer's. A group of inactive adults between twenty and sixty years of age was compared to more active peers. Researchers took into account all variables and still found that the risk of developing Alzheimer's in inactive people was four times that of active people.

There are several games in this book, but you can also find a myriad of puzzle books in your favorite bookstore. There are also a number of websites that offer games you can play online, and join others also playing the games. Why not have friends come over to play Scrabble or Bridge, and if you have to learn new skills, all the better!

"If you focus on results, you will never change. If you focus on change, you will get results."

—Jack Dixon

Increase Your Workout Intensity

Moderate-intensity exercise gets your heart pumping, but not in an overly stressful, breathless way. This kind of exercise helps you develop endurance. High-intensity exercise is tough; you breathe heavily and are overloading your heart and muscles. You need a mixture of both kinds of intensity to stay fit. When you push your intensity levels, your body responds by becoming stronger and burning more calories.

To improve your fitness level, you need to work your body harder than it is used to working, which means you need to overload or increase the intensity and/or duration of your exercise regimen. Research has found that your body adapts to the stress of working harder by becoming stronger. For example, if you walk 2 miles five days a week, eventually walking those 2 miles will get easier, and you'll be able to work longer or faster or both. Your heart becomes stronger and more efficient using this overload principle, but you can also apply this principle to the other components of physical fitness, including muscle strength, muscle endurance, and flexibility.

By systematically overloading your muscles in both strength and endurance (lifting more weight or lifting weight for longer), as well as in flexibility (stretching further and more extensively), you will also be able to make gains in those fitness elements. Lifting weights and stretching in a regular strengthening program allow you to create a body that is more capable and fitter than it was before. The harder you exercise, the higher the levels of both fat and sugar that you'll burn.

"By embracing your mother wound as your yoga, you transform what has been a hindrance in your life into a teacher of the heart."

—Phillip Moffitt

Stretch Your Back Muscles in Child's Pose

To do the child's pose (Balasana) kneel on all fours, with your hands under your shoulders and your knees under your hips. Inhale and on the exhalation draw your buttocks back to rest on your heels. Press your hands on the floor, extending into your fingertips, and stretching back through the sides of your body to the hips. Let your forehead rest on the floor. While in the pose, inhale, and feel the expansion of your waist and lower back. Exhale and observe the contraction of your ribs and lungs as the breath leaves your body. Stay for several breaths and then come back up and release the pose.

If your head does not reach the floor, place a folded blanket under the forehead. If your buttocks do not meet the heels, place a folded blanket between your heels and blanket for support. Walk your hands to the right for several breaths and then to the left. This stretches one side of the body at a time, and is particularly beneficial for scoliosis, where one side of the body is convex and the other is concave. The benefits of child's pose include the following:

- It increases circulation in the lower back and abdomen.
- It stretches the back muscles and the spine.
- It eases lower back discomfort.
- It's a good resting pose to do in between strenuous postures.

"There is nothing so American as our national parks."

—Franklin D. Roosevelt

Spend Your Saturday Supporting Our National Parks

Did you know that many of America's parks are in crisis with deteriorating roads, trails, and visitors' facilities? Some parks are operating without adequate funding. Pollution and traffic congestion exact a toll on these national treasures. If you live near, visit, or simply want to help a national park, here are three government websites you can visit to make a donation or volunteer your services:

- *www.nps.gov/getinvolved/donate.htm*
- *www.nationalparks.org/take-action/*
- *www.npca.org*

Your local parks also need help, as does the environment in general. Here are several ways you can improve your local outdoor environment:

- When you're enjoying public parks, keep an eye out for ways you can spruce them up. For instance, if you see litter don't just let it bother you; get out there and pick it up! Offer to plant flowers, shrubs, or trees.
- Adopt a bench at a local park. Use a plaque to memorialize your local company founder, or someone special on the job who has passed on. Attach the plaque to the bench's back support.
- Adopt a section of a highway. Keep it clean and beautiful. Organize a group to help you pick up trash along your designated section of the road. It goes a long way toward keeping America beautiful.

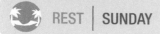

"The television, that insidious beast, that Medusa which freezes a billion people to stone every night, staring fixedly, that Siren which called and sang and promised so much and gave, after all, so little."

—Ray Bradbury, *The Golden Apples of the Sun*

Opt for Less Media Saturation

Digital cable, satellite dishes, streaming movies over the Internet, smartphones, MP3 hookups in the car, wireless Internet connections—ours is a technological world, and it can be pretty seductive. Some people can't resist the pleasure of watching a movie on their laptop while curled in bed, or having the highest of high-end stereo equipment, or exploring the world through the Internet for hours at a time. If you have a media habit, you certainly aren't alone. According to statistics compiled by a group called TV Free America, 98 percent of American households have at least one television, and 40 percent have three or more TVs! The television is turned on in the average American home for seven hours and twelve minutes every day, and 66 percent of Americans eat dinner while watching TV. Almost half of Americans (49 percent) admit they watch too much TV.

Like anything else, technology and media are fine . . . in moderation. But also, like anything else, too much of a good thing soon becomes a bad thing. If your media habit is taking up more than its fair share of your time and you are sacrificing other, equally important or more important parts of your life because of your media fixation, then it's a bad habit.

Seek balance in your media habits. Set boundaries. Don't let Internet surfing or channel surfing keep you from sleeping enough, eating right, or getting up out of your chair and getting some exercise.

"As a kid, I got three meals a day. Oatmeal,
miss-a-meal, and no meal."

—Mr. T.

Eat Oatmeal Often

Oatmeal is a marvelous choice for healthy fiber, both soluble and insoluble. Insoluble fiber slows down the digestion of starch, preventing a sharp rise in blood glucose levels after a meal. Soluble fiber aids in the processing and elimination of food, moving it quickly and efficiently through the bowels. Studies have shown that eating foods that are high in soluble fiber may help to lower LDL cholesterol (bad cholesterol) without lowering HDL cholesterol (good cholesterol). Whether you choose steel-cut oats (the most roughly cut and least processed), rolled or "old-fashioned" oats, quick oats, or instant, all types of oats are effective at reducing cholesterol. To get the daily 3 grams of soluble fiber recommended for lowering cholesterol levels, you'll need to eat 2 ounces of oat bran (²/₃ cup dry or about 1½ cups cooked) or 3 ounces of oatmeal (1 cup dry or 2 cups cooked). To increase the fiber benefits, add walnuts and raisins or fruits, such as blueberries or blackberries.

WEEK TWENTY-EIGHT

BASIC WHOLE-WHEAT PANCAKES

Serves 6
½ cup whole-wheat flour
¼ cup quick-cooking oatmeal
1 tablespoon Splenda
½ teaspoon baking powder
⅓ teaspoon baking soda
⅛ cup egg white substitute
1 cup skim milk
Add blueberries, bananas and pecans, cranberries and walnuts, or cinnamon and raisins to the batter before you cook the pancakes. Come up with fun toppings of your own.

BASIC WHOLE-WHEAT PANCAKES *continued*

1. In a bowl, mix all dry ingredients together. In a separate bowl, mix all wet ingredients together. Gently fold dry ingredients into wet ingredients.
2. Coat skillet or griddle with nonstick spray. Pour ⅓ cup batter per pancake onto skillet.
3. Cook on medium-high heat until pancake develops bubbles on top. Flip the pancake and brown on the other side.

PER SERVING: Calories 64 | **Fat** 0g | **Protein** 4g | **Sodium** 141mg | **Fiber** 2g | **Carbohydrates** 12g

"Another myth is that strength training is expensive, time consuming, and complex. In fact, it shouldn't take more than thirty minutes per session."

—James Peterson, PhD, sports medicine consultant

Add Lunges to Your Daily Workout

Lunges provide multiple benefits for your lower body, your legs, your inner and outer thighs, your hips, and your knees. There are three types of lunges that you can easily add to your daily workout. Complete an average of two to three sets with ten to twenty reps per set.

Stationary Lunge: Stand with feet hip width apart. Step one foot back, placing the ball of the foot on the floor. This is the starting position. Stabilize and balance in this position before moving into the lunge. Bend both knees to about 90 degrees (the back knee will almost touch the floor), then return to the starting position. If you find it hard to stay balanced, use a chair or wall to stabilize yourself throughout the movement. The motion should be straight down and up. With practice your balance will increase as will your lower body strength.

Reverse Lunge: Start with the feet hip width apart. Step one foot back and bend both knees about 90 degrees into a lunge. Using mostly the forward leg, pull yourself up to standing. Repeat this exercise with your opposite leg. This exercise builds strength and mobility in the hips as well as increases dynamic balance.

Lateral Lunge: Begin with your feet together and arms by your side. Step out to the right, bending the right knee and touching the left hand to the floor. Press off the right leg and bring the feet together. Repeat on the opposite side. Lateral Lunges strengthen the hips and inner and outer ligaments and tendons of the knees.

"We are never more fully alive, more completely ourselves, or more deeply engrossed in anything than when we are playing."

—Charles Schaefer

Stimulate Your Brain by Playing What's in a Name?

Find words using only the letters in a given name. Each letter in a name can be used only once in your word. For example, if the name is George Washington, then you could make the words *soar, grow, note,* and many others. Words that are always capitalized or require a hyphen or an apostrophe are not included in the answer lists. Words with variant or British spellings are also not included. Try this one:

Pablo Picasso

Find 10 five-letter words:

1. _____   6. _____
2. _____   7. _____
3. _____   8. _____
4. _____   9. _____
5. _____   10. _____

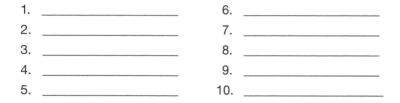

abaci, aboil, albas, alias, appal, apsis, aspic, assai, aspis, baals, bails, balas, basal, basic, basil, bassi, basso, bliss, blips, blocs, bloop, boils, bolas, bolos, cabal, capos, casas, cibol, claps, clasp, class, clips, clops, clops, cloops, coala, coals, cobia, coils, colas, coops, copal, isbas, labia, laics, lapis, lasso, lisps, lobos, locos, loops, oasis, obias, obolo, oboli, opals, opsio, ossia, opado, oilio, opobo, paces, pails, palpi, palps, papal, papas, pibal, pical, picas, pipal, pisco, pisos, plica, plops, polio, polis, polos, pools, posal, psoas, sails, slice, salps, salpa, salsa, scalp, scald, scoop, scops, sials, silos, silli, slabs, slaps, slips, slobs, sloop, slops, soaps, soils, solos, soPai, spail, spica, spics, spoil, spool

"As I've been able to once again gain the benefits of speed work, I'm enjoying my running more and more."

—Frank Shorter

Use Fartlek to Build Endurance

Fartlek, a Swedish word meaning "speed play," is an unstructured type of speed work. The central purpose of fartlek is to prepare you for the anaerobic demands that more structured speed workouts and racing provide. The primary purpose of including Fartlek in your regimen is to increase your anaerobic threshold to maintain a faster pace over longer periods of time. Basically, it builds your endurance by strengthening your body's ability to run longer and faster. You can run a fartlek workout at a fast pace in varying distances and durations—anywhere that's safe for running.

How to Practice Fartlek Running

Even though it is considered an unstructured workout, there are basic guidelines for fartlek running. Begin your workout with a minimum of 1–1½ miles of easy running (or a minimum of twelve minutes). End with a 1-mile cool-down, throw in speed bursts of varying times and distances, then follow each with a recovery jog.

The idea here is to practice running at a brisk effort (generally faster than your present 5K race pace), employing good running form and training your body to run anaerobically (meaning without oxygen). Push yourself until your breathing becomes labored and your pace begins to drop off. Rather than continuing to push yourself past this point (when you are running at a slow pace with deteriorating form due to fatigue), it's much more beneficial to run fast for a shorter period of time and then to resume when you recover (that is, catch your breath).

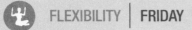
"Concentrating on poses clears the mind, while focusing on the breath helps the body shift out of fight-or-flight mode."

—Melanie Haiken, *Yoga Journal*, March 2006

Stretch Your Spine with Cat-Cow Pose

The cat-cow pose warms up the spine beautifully, creating suppleness and stretching the back muscles. Start on all fours, as a cat or cow would stand. Wrists are placed directly under shoulders and knees are placed directly under hips. Look forward and lengthen into the crown of the head and into the tailbone. Slightly tip the tailbone up. Inhale the breath. Press the inner thighs away from each other, hugging the bone. Exhale and round the spine by curling the chin into the chest and lifting each vertebrae up toward the ceiling. Draw the tailbone in between the legs toward the pubic bone. The pubic bone moves toward the navel and the navel recedes and presses up to the front of the spine. Press the hands down and push the hands away from the body as you round the back. Repeat the lengthening on the inhalation and rounding on the exhalation nine more times, coordinating the movement with the breath.

YOGA IS GOOD FOR YOUR HEART

In a recent study reported by *Yoga Journal,* a group of people who walked twenty minutes a day three times a week were compared to a group of yoga practitioners who did standing poses twenty minutes a day, three times a week. Guess who received the greater cardiovascular benefit? The yogis did!

"The primary conception of tennis is to get the ball over the net and at the same time to keep it within bounds of the court; failing this, within the borders of the neighborhood."

—Elliot Chaze

Play Tennis

Playing a game of tennis is a great way to get a workout, and you only need one other person to start a game of tennis. Playing tennis builds agility, hand-eye coordination, and works all the major muscle groups—and that helps your metabolism. Since the game is played in short bursts during which you're swinging your racquet or sprinting after a ball, it offers fat-burning benefits similar to those found in traditional interval training. A 150-pound individual can expect to burn more than 400 calories each hour and enjoy a competitive sport in the process.

As you play tennis, don't be surprised to find that not only are your tennis skills improving but your overall stamina, speed, coordination, agility, and flexibility are improving as well. According to Harvard's Dr. Ralph Paffenbarger, individuals who play at least three hours of tennis a week cut their risk of death from *any* cause by half. Maybe that alertness really does come in handy if there's a bus approaching.

Just remember to warm up your muscles first and take care to use proper hitting and serving techniques to prevent injuries. Tennis pros say that a couple of days each week on the court should be enough for a good workout.

IF YOU DON'T KNOW HOW TO PLAY, SIGN UP FOR LESSONS
Almost anyone, from eight- to ten-year-old children to seniors in their seventies or eighties, can play tennis. Lean how to play now and you can enjoy it for a lifetime. Plus, tennis is one of those games where you need another player. If you are playing doubles, you'll need three other players; so taking lessons is a good way to meet new people, get a workout, and feel great.

"I frequently tramped eight or ten miles through the deepest snow to keep an appointment with a beech-tree, or a yellow birch, or an old acquaintance among the pines."

—Henry David Thoreau

Make Time for Nature Outings

Studies show that spending time in nature promotes feelings of calm and relaxation. When you look at a beautiful sunset, enjoy the sounds of the pounding surf, or enjoy a beautiful view from the side of a mountain, the vastness of the world helps to put all the small frustrations back in the proper perspective. Find something active outside that you enjoy, and take time to put it in your schedule. You can incorporate nature with physical activity such as running, walking, or other activities and sports. Remember, regular physical activity is an important health behavior that can return multiple dividends. Not only will you feel better, look great, and manage your weight effectively, but you also will manage stress better by being active on a regular basis. Something as simple as a short walk can provide a powerful positive outlet for tension.

"Spinach is not only tasty, but it can help prevent osteoporosis, heart disease, colon cancer and arthritis. There have also been recent studies that suggest eating spinach may significantly lessen brain damage from strokes and other neurological disorders."

—Abby Kallio

Add Green Smoothies to Your Diet

Green smoothies are smoothies with greens blended into them. They differ from juices in that they're a complete food—they still have fiber. Most people know that greens are very nutritious, but struggle to eat enough of them—they're not the easiest vegetables to prepare tastefully while maintaining all of the important vitamins and minerals your body requires, and they can be hard to digest. Blended greens in smoothies have already been ripped apart and are effectively "predigested," allowing for almost immediate absorption. Also, the blending process used in green smoothies actually breaks down the cellulose in the greens, making the nutrients able to be absorbed 70 percent to 90 percent more than that of a traditional salad.

THE GREEN GO-GETTER

Packed with green spinach and apples, this creamy green smoothie will kick your morning off with a boost of essential amino acids, vitamins, minerals, and an absolutely amazing taste.

Recipe Yields: 3–4 cups
1 cup spinach
2 green apples, peeled and cored
1 banana, peeled
1 cup purified water

1. Combine spinach, apples, and banana with ½ cup of water in a blender and blend until thoroughly combined
2. Continue adding remaining water while blending until desired texture is achieved.

PER 1 CUP SERVING: Calories 89 | **Fat** 0g | **Protein** 1g | **Sodium** 10mg | **Fiber** 3g | **Carbohydrates** 23g

WEEK TWENTY-NINE

"Strength training is important to everyone, not only larger sized individuals, because we all need to be strong. And, it's possible to be thin and weak."

—Shirley S. Archer, fitness professional, Stanford University School of Medicine

Add Squats to Your Workout Routine

The squat is one of the most important exercises to maintain a healthy back, hips, and knees. And they are considered functional strength exercises because performing repetitions of them will increase your muscular strength and endurance. You perform movements very similar to squats all day long without even realizing it. Every time you sit down and stand up you are doing a squat—on and off of the couch, in and out of the car, up and down to use the restroom.

A basic squat is very similar to sitting down and standing up from a chair, which is a great way to begin learning a squat. Find a chair or stool that is close to the height of your knees. Stand with your back to the chair. Place your heels a few inches away from the base of the chair with your feet about a hip width apart or slightly wider. Start with your arms by your sides, and as you take your hips back and down, reach your arms forward to counterbalance your weight. Very lightly touch your hips to the seat and stand back up. Keep the pressure on the heels of your feet in order to make the back of the legs (hamstrings and gluts) do more work than the front of the legs (quads). Keep the pressure on your heels and elongate the spine; avoid letting your knees go beyond your toes.

In order to build a good combination of muscular strength and endurance, you should complete an average of two to three sets with ten to twenty reps per set. Once you have developed a solid squat position with a large range of motion, you can begin to speed up the repetitions of the squat.

"I love to roast vegetables that have been sprinkled with chopped ginger and olive oil. It really brings out the flavor of sweet potatoes and all kinds of squash."

—Nina Simonds

Feed Your Brain with a Ginger Citrus Smoothie

The tang of sweet citrus and the zing of ginger make for a stimulating blend that will get your senses and taste buds on high alert. With 4 servings of fruit and 2 servings of vegetables in this smoothie, the vitamin and mineral benefits are obvious, but this citrusy green mix is especially high in iron and folate. Necessary to optimal brain functioning, folate is especially important for pregnant and nursing women. Because this smoothie is delicious and rejuvenating, any stressful day can be turned around in no time by indulging in this treat!

GINGER CITRUS SMOOTHIE

Recipe Yields: 3–4 cups

1 cup watercress
2 cups pineapple, peeled and cored
2 bananas, peeled
¼" ginger, peeled
1 cup purified water

1. Combine watercress, pineapple, bananas, ginger, and ½ cup water in a blender and blend until thoroughly combined.
2. Add remaining ½ cup of water as needed while blending until desired consistency is achieved.

PER 1 CUP SERVING: Calories 91 | **Fat** 0g | **Protein** 1g | **Sodium** 6mg | **Fiber** 2g | **Carbohydrates** 23g

"Individuals who engage in sixty minutes of exercise per day may need as much as 6 to 10 grams of carbohydrates per kilogram of body weight per day."

—Tina Angelotti, developer of the Krav Maga fitness program

Eat More Carbs to Fuel Endurance Training

Just like a car needs gasoline to continue to run, your body needs fuel in the form of food. If you owned a Lamborghini Diablo, you would likely recoil at the idea of fueling it with a low-grade gasoline, something that could cause the engine to seize up. Think of your body the same way. When undergoing endurance training, in particular, you need to choose high-quality fuel for your body to run efficiently.

Carbohydrates are a major source of fuel for the body, particularly when participating in endurance training. Glucose is the primary source of energy in most cells, and it's produced in your body from the carbohydrates you eat. If you don't eat enough carbs to generate the glucose levels needed to keep up with the energy demands of endurance training, your body will be forced to make glucose from your muscle proteins. Not all carbs are equal, so here's a list of the healthiest carb choices:

- Brown rice
- Sweet potato
- All fruits
- All vegetables
- Yams
- Whole-wheat pasta
- Brown rice pasta

- Soba noodles
- Beans
- Lentils
- Whole-wheat bread
- Whole-grain bread
- Whole-wheat couscous
- Quinoa

"An instructor once told me that when there's resistance in your body, it's only because of the resistance in your mind. It's about getting inside the pose. Being the breath."

—Lisa Bonet

Strengthen Your Upper Back Muscles with the Sphinx Pose

Lie on your belly with your legs extended behind you. Prop yourself up on your forearms. Your forearms will be parallel to each other with the elbows close to the waist and in line with the wrists and shoulders. Press the forearms and the palms down and observe how this grounding action lifts your chest and elongates the sides of your body. Maintaining this action, pull your elbows back on the floor without actually moving them. Feel the muscles of the upper back draw in to the back and hug your shoulder blades. Enhance this by lifting your sternum forward and up. Enjoy the openness and broadness of the top chest. Stay for several breaths and then release down and rest.

The benefits of the sphinx pose include the following:

- It strengthens the upper back muscles.
- It opens the chest and stretches the muscles on the front body.
- It teaches basic back-bending action.

YOGA IS MIRACULOUS!

Dr. Benjamin Spock was a guru to parents for many generations. During the last years of his life, doctors told him he would never be able to walk again. Instead of resigning himself to that fate, Spock began a regimen of macrobiotics, shiatsu massage, psychoanalysis, and yoga. After four yoga classes with a master, he was able to walk again.

---

*"Take your victories, whatever they may be, cherish them,
use them, but don't settle for them."*

—Mia Hamm

Play Soccer or Other Outdoor Activities with Your Family

When your children are old enough to run around, get out a soccer ball and take it to the yard or park. Children love to participate in activities with their parents. Whether or not you realize it, you are teaching your child even as you play games with him. As you demonstrate a competitive spirit, team cooperation, respect for the rules of the game, and good sportsmanship whether you win or lose, he learns through observation, listening, and participation. So go outside and run around with your kids. If soccer isn't your thing, make up a game. The point is to play, set a good example, and have fun with the little (or not so little) ones in your life. Compare the following list of activities and choose your game accordingly.

• Reading or watching TV burns 75 calorie per hour.
• Playing softball or soccer burns 260 calories per hour.
• Playing football, hockey, or basketball burns 460 calories per hour.

LET YOUR CHILD LEAD THE WAY

Children are expert in the art of play, and they are natural-born teachers. If you are feeling stressed out, overworked, doggedly tired, take a timeout for play. It strengthens the parent/child bond. Don't remember how? Playing with your baby or toddler can get you laughing, relieve stress, increase spontaneity, and inspire creativity. You probably don't require a child development expert to explain to you what floor time is. Get down on the same level as your youngster and give your full attention to him or her. Permit your child to lead the way for your own inner child to come out.

"I am thankful for laughter except when milk comes out of my nose."

—Woody Allen

Eat Foods Containing Tryptophan (5-HTP) to Improve Sleep

The body makes a chemical known as 5-HTP from the tryptophan we get from food. The 5-HTP used in supplements comes from the seeds of an African plant *(Griffonia simplicifolia)*. In our bodies, 5-HTP quickly becomes serotonin, a neurotransmitter (a chemical that carries messages to and from the brain) that affects sleep cycles, appetite, and mood. Extra tryptophan in our diets leads to extra serotonin in our brains, which is why the supplements are touted as a sleep aid and mood-lifter, among other things.

Foods that provide tryptophan (5-HTP) include roasted white turkey, ground beef, cottage cheese, chicken thighs, eggnog, milk, and almonds.

"At the age of 61, I feel and look great (so I'm told!), have good bone density, and enjoy general good health. Genes play a part, no doubt, but I can't help but give some credit to my soy-rich diet."

—Brita Housez, *Tofu Mania: Add Tofu to 120 of Your Favorite Dishes*

Make It a Tofu Day

Tofu (soybean curd) is a marvelous source of protein—and it's cholesterol-free, contains no saturated fat, is a great source of fiber, contains calcium, vitamin E, and B vitamins, and is rich in the two polyunsaturated fats essential to optimal health. Here's a simple, yet delicious way to add tofu to your diet:

ASIAN SOUP WITH TOFU

Serves 4
1 package firm tofu, cubed
1 cup shiitake mushrooms, soak in water for 25 to 30 minutes before cooking, remove stems, and slice.
½ cup canned bamboo shoots, drained and sliced
½ cup canned water chestnuts, drained and sliced
3 cups low-sodium chicken broth
1 tablespoon rice wine
1 tablespoon low-sodium soy sauce
1 teaspoon sesame oil
2 tablespoons rice vinegar
1 teaspoon ground ginger
½ cup green onions, sliced

Add all ingredients to a saucepan and bring to a boil. Simmer for 15 minutes.

"Squat more."

—Jesse Marunde

Add a Somo Squat to Your Routine

This variation of a squat is easier to learn for many people. It may also be a better choice for people with chronic knee pain. The feet are placed wide and the toes are turned out about 45 degrees. (It's fine if your angle is a little more than 45 degrees.) The torso stays upright as the knees bend over the big and second toes. The hips will not travel back nearly as much for this kind of squat. The pressure is still primarily on the heel of the foot in the upward as well as the downward phase. You may hold a hand weight or a ball to increase the resistance. This exercise is a great way to strengthen, lengthen, as well as open the hips and the inner musculature of the legs.

"I was starting to become impotent through this diet [all fast food for thirty days] and couldn't perform. How many people who are taking the little blue pill, if they started to change what they are eating most of the time, could change the way their sex life is?"

—Morgan Spurlock, *Supersize Me*

Don't Mix Chronic Stress with a High-Fat Diet

Researchers at the James A. Haley Veterans Administration Medical Center, at the University of South Florida (USF), and Arizona State University (ASU) found that chronically stressed rats consuming an "American-style" diet of excessive carbohydrates and beef fat developed atrophy in the hippocampus, the part of the brain that is essential for learning and remembering new information. Rats fed a high-fat diet and living under chronic stress (living in crowded conditions, in close proximity to cats) developed hippocampal atrophy, expressed in reduced dendrite length. Dendrites are the connections between brain cells where information is stored. The researchers deduced that the combination of a high-fat diet and stress could interfere with the ability of the brain—in rats or people—to learn new information. Previous research had shown that rats on a high-fat diet produce an excessive amount of corticosterone in response to stress. Corticosterone, a steroid hormone produced by the adrenal glands, can also damage the hippocampus, indicating that a high-fat diet and stress are doubly detrimental to the brain.

"I have always struggled to achieve excellence. One thing that cycling has taught me is that if you can achieve something without a struggle it's not going to be satisfying."

—Greg LeMond

Add Cycling to Enhance Your Running Performance

Cycling exercises some of the same muscle groups as running, such as the quadriceps and shins, both of which don't develop as rapidly from workouts as the calf muscles and hamstrings. Cycling also strengthens the connective tissue of the knee, hip, and ankle regions, thus reducing the risk of injury. After a stressful run, cycling can loosen fatigued leg muscles.

There are three types of biking to try: road riding; mountain biking; and stationary cycling. Taking place on the road, road biking allows you to travel long distances with speed. Mountain bikes are two-wheel, all-terrain vehicles that can be ridden almost anywhere. Although mountain biking is a lot of fun and challenging, its jarring nature makes falls risky. Road and stationary cycling are better alternatives. With stationary cycling, you can work out indoors year-round regardless of inclement weather. Stationary cycling offers the additional benefit of being able to safely listen to music or read while working out.

A few things to keep in mind: Refrain from cycling on a scheduled rest day. Since it's much more difficult to run after cycling, run prior to heading out on your bike. Spin easily, as opposed to grinding big gears. Be sure that your seat height and pedals are properly positioned. Finally, always wear a helmet, and leave the iPod at home!

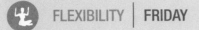

"Anyone who practices can obtain success in yoga but not one who is lazy. Constant practice alone is the secret of success."

—Svatmarama, Hatha Yoga Pradipika

Limber Up Your Spine with the Cobra Pose

To do the cobra pose (Bhujangasana), lie on your belly with your forehead on the floor, your hands under your shoulders, and your legs outstretched (together) behind you. Press your hands and the front of your feet down and lengthen your toes away from your body. Draw your elbows into the waist. Inhale the breath and look forward. Feel the breath ease as your chest opens. Stretch your chest, the area between your shoulder blades (upper back), and your ribs forward. Your ribs and the belly move away from your hips and your hips stretch away from the legs. The pubic bone remains on the floor and the lower back and tailbone lengthen away from the upper body. Space is created between your hips and your ribs, allowing your spine to lengthen into your body. Your belly receives a pleasant stretch. Make sure you exhale completely.

Next, coil your spine into your body, like a wave that is moving in and up to arc before it spills over into the surf. Use your hands pressing down to lengthen your arms up to support the coiling action of your spine. Your arms do not have to straighten and they should not be used to create a pushup feeling (which will cause shortening of your lower back and compression). Breathe! Come up only as far as is comfortable. Stay in the pose for a few breaths and then come down. Repeat several times.

The benefits of the cobra pose include the following:

- It stretches the front side of the body and its organs.
- It strengthens the spine and back muscles.
- It relieves backache.
- When done correctly, it can relieve sciatica and slipped disc (best done under the supervision of a qualified yoga professional).

"Never doubt that a small group of committed people can change the world. Indeed, it is the only thing that ever has."

—Margaret Mead

Take a Volunteer Vacation

Want to go abroad but don't want to spend your days fighting through crowds of tourists or lying idle on a beach? Consider taking a volunteer vacation where you can provide valuable service, while simultaneously seeing new sights. Many do involve travel costs, but they also offer unique experiences, new friendships, and a chance to energize yourself through performing service. Here are two international organizations than can help you find opportunities and plan your trip:

1. Global Volunteers (*www.globalvolunteers.com*)
2. International Volunteer Programs Association (*www.volunteer international.org*)

There are, of course, volunteer vacation opportunities in America, as well. Several national organizations that offer information about volunteer vacations include:

- *www.volunteerguide.org*
- *www.sierraclub.org/outings/national/service.aspx*
- *www.americanhiking.org*

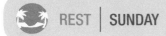

"Yoga is bodily gospel."

—Reaven Fields

Try Yoga Meditation as a Path to Unitive Consciousness

Yoga provides a powerful tool for reducing tension and stress and for bringing you back in touch with your true self and your inner reality. In yoga meditation, you learn to slow down long enough to observe the workings of your mind and emotions, and to realize the preciousness of the present moment. When you practice yoga meditation, it helps you put things that once seemed earth shattering into perspective, to become more conscious of your thought patterns, the vacillation of your emotions, and how you can approach them in new ways.

Yoga meditation also offers you a path to understanding and owning your innate intelligence. New thoughts and ways of being emerge. (The body is also learning new patterns of movement through the practice of yoga postures.) You discover that what is happening in your mind permeates every cell in your body. With dutiful practice, you learn to unify your mind-body system and experience the realization of oneness and unity with all other beings, known as *unitive consciousness.*

This is a material world, where external achievement and the accumulation of wealth in the form of money and possessions are the main measure of success and the American Dream. Greed and excessive consumption is rampant. Computers and television passively entertain and isolate. Immediate gratification appears to be at our fingertips. Unfortunately, this route leads to alienation from your real, internal self, with the resultant feelings of emptiness and apathy. The practice of yoga meditation can help fill this void by offering a path to inner fulfillment and spirituality.

*"If I could eat only one food for the rest of my life,
it would definitely be beans."*

—Cynthia Sass, RD

Fall In Love with Beans

Beans are so jam-packed with nutrients that they qualify as both a vegetable and a protein. That's kind of like being both king and queen! A cup of beans provides a whopping 13 grams of fiber (half of our daily requirement), about 15 grams of protein, and dozens of key nutrients, including calcium, potassium, and magnesium. Eating 3 cups of beans every week is recommended. By the way, it's okay to buy canned beans, as rinsing them for one minute in cold water will wash away a quarter of the sodium. However, when you do buy canned beans, here are two primary suggestions:

- **Buy low-sodium beans**: If you're watching your salt intake (and you should be), purchase canned low-sodium beans. Once you use the cold water trick, you've significantly decreased the amount of salt you're ingesting.
- **Buy vegetarian beans**: Baked and refried varieties are traditionally prepared with lard or pork, which add calories, cholesterol, sodium, and saturated fat, none of which you want to add into your diet. A healthier alternative is vegetarian refried beans. They contain no saturated fat and have 2 more grams of protein than the nonvegetarian ones.

WEEK THIRTY-ONE

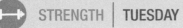

"More weight with less reps builds strength, and less weight with more reps builds endurance. You should train for both strength and endurance."

—Jeff Levine, Krav Maga instructor

Do Your Squats While Holding a Ball

Once you've mastered the basic squat, adding a ball can amp up the workout. Basically, squatting with a ball works the same muscles in the lower body as a basic squat. The only difference is that you hold a medicine ball in your hands as you squat. (If you don't have a medicine ball, you can use hand weights or even a basketball or soccer ball.) As you drop down into the squat, touch the ball lightly to the floor. As you come up from your squat take the ball up over your head, extending through the entire length of your body. Concentrate on controlling both the upward and the downward motions in order to build stability of the exercise. This exercise develops muscular strength in the lower body and the upper body simultaneously. It also emphasizes a great deal of the muscles in your trunk.

In order to build a good combination of muscular strength and endurance, you should complete an average of two to three sets with 10–20 reps per set. Use a weight that leaves you feeling some fatigue by the time you've completed about twelve repetitions. If you complete twenty repetitions with a 6-pound ball and you can do another ten reps, it's time to start using a heavier ball!

HOW HEAVY SHOULD THE BALL BE?

If you are a beginner, start with a ball such as a handball, basketball, or soccer ball before progressing to a weighted ball. When using a weighted ball, the recommended starting weight for women is 4 pounds and for men at least 6–8 pounds. If you do not have a weighted ball, a hand weight will work just as well.

"A vigorous five-mile walk will do more good for an unhappy but otherwise healthy adult than all the medicine and psychology in the world."

—Paul Dudley White

De-Stress Through Exercise

Stress evokes the "fight or flight" reaction by releasing stress hormones into the body designed to give us sudden, quick reactions, extra strength, and endurance. When we don't respond to the stress response by moving quickly, using our strength, or taking advantage of the added endurance, muscles stay tense, blood pressure stays high, breathing stays shallow, and all that cortisol and adrenaline course through the body causing all kinds of problems.

Exercise changes the picture, accomplishing two important things in the wake of the stress response:

1. Exercise allows the body to expend energy so that while your brisk walk around the block may not actually be "fight or flight," to the body, the message is the same. That extra energy available to your body is being used, signaling the body that it can, after exercise, return to equilibrium.
2. Exercise also releases chemicals like beta endorphins that specifically counteract the effects of stress hormones, alerting the body that the danger has passed and the relaxation response can begin.

Yoga, Pilates, stretching, and other mind-body exercises relax the mind as well as the body by helping link movement to the breath, which, in turn, stops the physical response to stress. These gentle levels of activity can burn off the physical tension, relax your muscles, and, at the same time, keep your worrying brain from obsessing about a concern for too long.

"Sooner or later a rider will emerge who will win more Tours. In every sport we have seen how the records eventually get broken and cycling is no exception."

—Miguel Indurain

Cycle Up Hills to Boost Endurance

Riding your bicycle on hills is similar to weight training, and adds a lot of leg strength. If you haven't done a lot of riding, you may be surprised at how tough it is to negotiate a hill on a bicycle. As with all other new activities, start slowly. With each workout, however, it will get easier, and your confidence will grow.

On days when the weather interferes with your bike training, you can get a good workout on a stationary bike at your fitness center or at home. All stationary bikes indicate mileage and calories burned, and many have programs that simulate hills and other variables. It's not exactly the same as your regular ride, but it's a great alternative when it's raining outside or if the roads are iced over.

Another indoor option is a fluid trainer, a stationary platform that your bike sits on that allows the rear wheel to rotate as you pedal. You can adjust the resistance as you go to simulate a variable terrain.

SHRUG OFF BAD DAYS

As with training for any sport or endeavor, there will be days when things just don't go well: Everything seems to be a struggle, or fatigue overtakes you sooner than you expected. You can't let these minor setbacks get you down. Learning to shrug off the bad workouts instead of obsessing about them is part of your growth as an athlete.

"Vogue and Self are putting out the message of yoginis as buff and perfect. If you start doing yoga for those reasons, fine. Most people get beyond that and see that it's much, much more."

—Patricia Walden

Wring Out Your Body with Stomach-Turning Twists

To do the stomach-turning pose (Jathara Parivartanasana) lie down on your back and bend your knees, placing your feet flat on the floor. Lift your feet away from the floor, bringing your knees to your chest. Extend your arms horizontally out to the sides on the floor. Stack your knees and ankles and let your knees come down to the right, toward the floor at a right angle. Your legs will hover over the floor, with your lower leg holding up your upper leg. Gaze up at the ceiling. Feel your belly and ribs spiral toward the left. Maintain the length of your spine upon inhalation, twist on the exhalation, and roll your left shoulder down toward the floor (without forcing). Stay in the pose for several breaths, deepening the twist. Then, bring your knees back to center and go to the other side. If hip mobility is restricted or your lower back is weak, place a folded blanket under the bottom leg for support.

The benefits of stomach-turning twists include the following:

- It is a powerful, stimulating, and wringing action for the waist, abdomen, and lower back.
- It strengthens transverse and oblique abdominal muscles.
- It strengthens inner and outer thigh muscles.

YOUR HEAD SHOULD FOLLOW, NOT LEAD

When twisting, do not let your head lead the way. There is a tendency to want to see where you're going, so the head and the eyes get overzealous. Twists spiral your spine and the body from the bottom up, like a corkscrew. Your head is the last to turn and it learns from the chest.

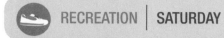

"Live in the sunshine, swim the sea, drink the wild air."

—Ralph Waldo Emerson

Go Swimming

Oh, go jump in a lake. No, really. Swimming is one of the best exercises you can do. It provides a total-body workout but is also low-impact so it won't hurt your joints as it improves stamina and flexibility. The water buoys the body so that joints, bones, and muscles don't feel the impact of exercise, making injuries less likely for people who are vulnerable to the impact. Work up gradually to thirty to sixty minutes of steady swimming. Varying your strokes—freestyle, breaststroke, backstroke, sidestroke—will help work all your muscles.

Although your maximum heart rate may be up to 30 beats lower when you're working out in the water, you're still burning a significant amount of calories and your lungs are taking in more oxygen than if you were resting and that helps burn fat.

If you already know how to swim but feel like you are treading water more than swimming, a few lessons can make the difference between frustration and enjoyment, as well as increase the effectiveness of your workouts. Your local fitness club or YMCA likely offers adult swimming lessons, and many cities offer swimming lessons through adult-education programs.

SIGN UP FOR WATER AEROBICS

Water aerobics is very popular and fun, too. Water aerobics can be tailored to any fitness level. Check your local pool or health club for water aerobics classes. Some areas even offer water yoga classes!

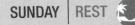

"I don't fear death because I don't fear anything I don't understand. When I start to think about it, I order a massage and it goes away."

—Hedy Lamarr

Get a Warm Rose Oil Massage

A massage is a great way to release the stress and tension you hold in your body. There's nothing comparable to human touch coupled with aromatherapy to transport you into a place of relaxation and peace. If you don't like rose scent, ask the masseuse to use sandalwood, ylang ylang, myrrh, or your favorite essential oil. Massages are de rigeur at day spas. They are also offered at deeply discounted rates at local colleges with massage therapy training programs. Another option is to ask your significant other to give you a massage, but be advised that making that choice could lead to other activities. Ah, but that could also relieve stress and put a smile on your face.

"After-dinner talk/Across the walnuts and the wine."

—Alfred, Lord Tennyson

Eat a Handful of Nuts

Nuts are high in fat, but they contain minerals, fiber, and nice amounts of protein. All nuts and seeds are small powerhouses. They are so powerful, in fact, that just having a serving of nuts five times a week can significantly reduce your risk for heart disease. However, nuts are high in calories and should be eaten in moderation; think of a serving as a tablespoon or two. Look for nuts that are unsalted; it's not important whether they are roasted or unroasted. Nuts are great sprinkled on foods high in vitamin C, such as fruit and vegetables, because the vitamin C increases the body's absorption of the iron in nuts.

WEEK THIRTY-TWO

"Strength training will build that essential lean body mass to rev up your metabolism and help stop those extra pounds from creeping on."

—Shirley S. Archer, fitness professional, Stanford University School of Medicine

Add Diagonal Reaches and Rotations to Your Squats with a Ball

Once you've mastered squats while holding a ball, you can easily add diagonal reaches and rotations to strengthen even more muscles.

For diagonal reaches: As you go down in the squat, rotate your torso to the right side, reaching the ball down at a 45-degree angle. As you come up, bring the ball back up diagonally across your body at a 45-degree angle to the left. Be sure to perform the same amount of repetitions on both sides. This exercise builds strength in the lower, middle, and upper body as well as strengthens the ligaments and tendons on the inner and outer knee.

For rotations: Place your feet further apart with the toes turned out slightly. Come to the bottom of your squat and hold it. That is the static part. Holding a ball with your arms stretched out in front of you, rotate your torso right and left. Your eyes will follow the direction the ball goes. This builds muscular endurance in your lower body and increases dynamic strength in your trunk. It also develops stability in the inner and outer ligaments and tendons of your knee.

Complete an average of two to three sets with ten to twenty reps per set, and if the exercises become too easy, use a heavier ball and adjust your reps as needed. To keep upping your muscular strength, increase the weight of the ball over time, and speed up your repetitions.

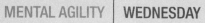

"The art of simplicity is a puzzle of complexity."

—Doug Horton

Tease Your Brain with Word Ladders

Link these word pairs together with a ladder of words. Each step in the ladder must be a real word and must differ from the previous word by only one letter. For example, CAT can be linked to DOG with these steps: CAT, COT, DOT, DOG. There are many possible solutions for these puzzles, but try to use only the given number of steps.

WATER to PALES (six steps)

_____   _____

OUTER to BAKED (seven steps)

_____   _____

TIGER to MATED (eight steps)

_____   _____

"You have a choice. You can throw in the towel, or you can use it to wipe the sweat off of your face."

—Gatorade advertisement

Try a Smoothie That's a Cyclist's Best Friend

Nothing keeps sustained energy up like slow-releasing carbohydrates. Root vegetables are the best friend of any distance cyclist on a mission for better times and better health!

CARBOHYDRATE BOOSTER

Recipe Yields: 3–4 cups

1 cup spinach
2 yams, peeled (microwave for two minutes, if softening is needed)
2 apples, peeled and cored
2 carrots, peeled
2 cups purified water

1. Combine spinach, yams, apples, carrots, and 1 cup water in a blender and blend until thoroughly combined.
2. Add remaining 1 cup water as needed while blending until desired consistency is achieved.

PER 1 CUP SERVING: Calories 110 | **Fat** 0g | **Protein** 2g | **Sodium** 50mg | **Fiber** 4g | **Carbohydrates** 27g

---

WHY ATHLETES EAT FRUIT

The recommended diet for athletes includes lots of fruits and vegetables, which might seem to be a contradiction because many fruits contain fructose, a simple sugar. These are natural sources of carbohydrates, and are low in simple sugar, and they contain fiber, which slows down the absorption of the sugar. Foods with added sugar are the ones to avoid.

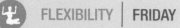

"Before you've practiced, the theory is useless. After you've practiced, the theory is obvious."

—David Williams

Make Your Spine Supple with a Sage Twist

To do a sage twist (Bharadvajasana) sit sideways on a chair. The right side of the body is next to the back of the chair. Plant your feet flat on the floor with heels under knees. If your feet do not reach the floor, bring the floor to you by placing a book or two under your feet.

Hold onto the topsides of the chair back and bend the elbows wide apart to stretch and open your rib cage, making more room for the breath to enter. Press your buttock bones down into the chair seat as you inhale and lengthen the sides of the body up. Exhale and gradually revolve the body around the spine, toward the back of the chair. With every inhalation, create lift, extension, and space in the body. After three or four breaths carefully unwind and return to center. Repeat on the other side. The benefits of the sage twist on chair include the following:

- It relieves arthritis of the lower back.
- It improves digestion.
- It alleviates rheumatism of the knees.
- It tones the liver and kidneys.
- It increases circulation to the abdominal organs.
- It exercises the abdominal muscles.
- It increases suppleness of spinal muscles.

"For instance, the bicycle is the most efficient machine ever created: Converting calories into gas, a bicycle gets the equivalent of three thousand miles per gallon."

—Bill Strickland, *The Quotable Cyclist*

Go for a Bike Ride

Riding a bike is a great way to get a hard workout in a short amount of time. You can ride indoors and out. Of course, riding outside will give you lots of fresh air, which will help you feel healthy and refreshed. If you are riding again for the first time in a long time, do so in an area where you can relax and familiarize yourself with the gearing and braking systems. They may seem complicated at first, but once you understand how they work, you'll breeze right through them. Your body will initially have to adjust to cycling, so limit your first few rides to shorter periods of time and build up to longer rides gradually.

WHAT'S THE DIFFERENCE BETWEEN ROAD BIKING AND MOUNTAIN BIKING?

Road biking takes place on the road, and allows you to travel long distances with speed. Mountain biking is more technical and requires a sense of adventure and a secure sense of balance. Although the name implies it, mountain bike riding does not mean you are limited to riding on mountains. To ensure you have the proper frame size and fit on a bike, talk to your local bike-store expert or bike club. As far as seat positioning goes, your knees should have a slight bend (15 to 20 degrees) when you are in the down phase of the pedal stroke, and your hips should not sway from side to side when you pedal.

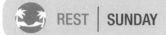

"That the birds of worry and care fly over your head, this you cannot change, but that they build nests in your hair, this you can prevent."

—Chinese Proverb

Curb Worrywart Tendencies

Are you a worrywart? How many of the following describe you?

- You find yourself worrying about things that are extremely unlikely, such as suffering from a freak accident or developing an illness you have no reason to believe you would develop. (Think Woody Allen and his imaginary brain tumor.)
- You have trouble falling asleep because you can't slow down your frantic worrying process as you lie still in bed at night.
- When the phone rings or the mail arrives, you immediately imagine what kind of bad news you are about to receive.
- You feel compelled to control the behaviors of others because you worry that they can't take care of themselves.
- You are overly cautious about engaging in any behavior that could possibly result in harm or hurt to you or to those around you, even if the risk is small (such as driving a car, flying in an airplane, or visiting a big city).

If even just one of the worrywart characteristics describes you, you probably worry more than you have to. Worry and the anxiety it can produce can cause specific physical, cognitive, and emotional symptoms, from heart palpitations, dry mouth, hyperventilation, muscle pain, and fatigue to fear, panic, anger, and depression. Make a list, right now, of ten things you can do to reduce your stress. Also, list all those worries and then assess the real possibility that each will come to pass. Often we worry needlessly, and life is just too short!

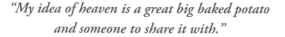
*"My idea of heaven is a great big baked potato
and someone to share it with."*

—Oprah Winfrey

Eat a Sweet Potato Instead of Broccoli

Sweet potatoes have high amounts of beta carotene, equal to that of carrots; and for 90 calories per sweet potato you get a huge amount of health-building nutrients. Beta carotene is a major fighter against cancer, heart disease, asthma, and rheumatoid arthritis. The bright orange flesh of the sweet potato contains carotenoids that help stabilize your blood sugar and lower insulin resistance, making cells more responsive to insulin, and aiding your metabolism. Sweet potatoes have four times the USRDA for beta carotene when eaten with the skin on. In fact, it would take 20 cups of broccoli to provide the 38,000 IUs of beta carotene (vitamin A) available in one cup of cooked sweet potatoes. They are a source of vitamin E, vitamin B_6, potassium, and iron, plus they're fat-free. Cup for cup, sweet potatoes have been found to provide as much fiber as oatmeal. Here's a great soup recipe to try:

RED LENTIL AND SWEET POTATO SOUP

Serves 4
1 white onion, chopped
1 celery stick, finely chopped
1 large carrot, sliced
1½ cups sweet potato, cubed
1 cup red lentils
1 bay leaf
½ teaspoon fresh garlic, minced
½ teaspoon all-purpose seasoning
5 cups vegetable or chicken broth
2 tablespoons fresh cilantro, chopped

RED LENTIL AND SWEET POTATO SOUP *continued*

1. In large saucepan, add onions and celery and cook on medium-high heat for 2 minutes, stirring often.
2. Add carrots, sweet potatoes, lentils, bay leaf, garlic, all-purpose seasoning, and broth to saucepan. Cover and cook on medium for 10 minutes.
3. Simmer for an additional 10 minutes. Remove bay leaf and blend soup in batches in a food processor.
4. Return soup to saucepan, add cilantro, and simmer for 5 minutes.

PER SERVING: Calories 289 | **Fat** 2g | **Protein** 21g | **Sodium** 1,033mg | **Fiber** 18g | **Carbohydrates** 47g

"So many older people, they just sit around all day long and they don't get any exercise. Their muscles atrophy, and they lose their strength, their energy, and vitality by inactivity."

—Jack LaLanne

Add a Medicine Ball Squat with Overhead Toss

When you have improved your squats and your arm strength, you can add to your basic squats with a medicine ball in a couple of ways. One is by tossing the ball into the air and catching it, and another is to toss the ball against a wall. Here's how to do it:

1. While holding the medicine ball at the height of your chin, drop down into a basic squat.
2. As you come up, toss the ball straight over your head as high as you can.
3. Catch the ball with your arms extended away from you.
4. Bend your arms to bring the ball back to chin level as you bend into your next squat.

For the second variation, squat down the same way but throw the ball up high against a wall, absorbing the downward force of the ball as you catch it.

Obviously, it's very important to keep your eyes on the ball for the duration of these exercises. You don't want it to land on your head, or to lose control of it. If it feels too strenuous, ease your way into it by going slowly and only tossing the ball a few inches at a time.

If you have a medicine ball that bounces, you can also reach the ball over your head then slam it down as you squat. Or you can bounce it to a partner, against a wall, or just catch it yourself.

*"What you see before you, my friend, is the result
of a lifetime of chocolate."*

—Katharine Hepburn

Treat Your Brain to Chocolate

In a study done by Salk Institute researcher Henriette van Praag and colleagues, a compound found in cocoa, epicatechin, combined with exercise, was found to promote functional changes in a part of the brain involved in the formation of learning and memory. Epicatechin is one of a group of chemicals called flavonols, which have previously been shown to improve cardiovascular function and increase blood flow to the brain. Dr. van Praag's findings, published in the May 30, 2007, issue of *The Journal of Neuroscience*, suggest a diet rich in flavonoids could help reduce the effects of neurodegenerative illnesses such as Alzheimer's disease or cognitive disorders related to aging.

FOR MAXIMUM BENEFIT, CHOOSE DARK CHOCOLATE

According to study results published in the American Chemical Society's *Journal of Agriculture and Food Chemistry,* cocoa powder has nearly twice the antioxidants in red wine and up to three times what is found in green tea. Based on the U.S. Department of Agriculture / American Chemical Society's findings, dark chocolate tested the highest for antioxidants over other fruits and vegetables. Comparing the levels of antioxidants dark chocolate came in with a score of 13,120; its closest competitor, milk chocolate, had levels of 6,740, and third was prunes at 5,770. The best source for healthy chocolate is raw, organic chocolate and the best outcome is to eat one or two small squares a few times a week, as it is, unfortunately, a tad fattening.

"The reason Armstrong has become the world's most indomitable cyclist and America's greatest athlete is two-pronged: He has both the physiology and the passion for his chosen vocation. . . . The more Lance hurts [and] the more wasted he becomes, the happier he is."

—Rob Fernas

Add Drills to Your Cyling Workouts

A lot of riding will develop endurance, but there are specific drills that can improve your technique and strength. Here are a few useful drills to consider.

- **One-legged drill.** On a stationary cycle with stirrups to keep your feet in place, pedal with one leg for about thirty seconds, then shift to the other leg and do the same. Repeat this drill three to five times.
- **Spinup.** Typically done outside, although you can do it indoors. During your ride, hunker down in the seat so that you don't bounce and quickly increase your revolutions per minute to 110. Hold that pace for one minute, then cool down for as long as you need to before starting the next. Do this five times during one ride, once a week.
- **Gear shifts.** This drill should be outside too, but you could do it on an indoor trainer. While riding, shift to a harder gear—one that makes you drop from 90 rpm to between 70 and 80—and stay with it for one or two minutes. Repeat five or six times. This drill simulates hills, so if you regularly ride in a hilly area, you can achieve the same result by pushing hard when you climb hills. You can also simulate hill climbing by changing to a harder gear and standing up to pedal for about thirty seconds at a time.
- **Time trial.** Find yourself a long, safe stretch of road and push your workout for approximately 10 miles (roughly thirty minutes). Do this drill once every couple of weeks. Do the time trials on the same course so that you can see how you are progressing.

"Mountain pose teaches us, literally, how to stand on our own two feet . . . teaching us to root ourselves into the earth. . . . Our bodies become a connection between heaven and earth."

—Carol Krucoff

Improve Your Agility with the Mountain Pose

The mountain pose (Tadasana) is the basic standing pose. Start by placing your feet together, joining the big toes and inner ankles. When viewed from one side, your ear, shoulder, hip, knee, and ankle should form a straight, vertical line, with your arms by your sides. Create your yoga feet by spreading the toes and balls of the feet, pressing into the big and little toe mounds, and the center of your heel. Bring the weight a little more into your heels. Lift your arches as you ground your feet. Enhance this action by lengthening your leg muscles all the way up to your hips. Lift the top of your kneecaps up by contracting your quadricep muscle. Firm the muscles of your thigh to the bone. Now you have created a strong and stable base from which your torso will be able to extend. This is like creating the mantle for the mountain to rise out of. Place your hands on your hips and extend the sides of the body from your hips to your armpits. This action creates length and space in the spine. Bring your arms back to your sides without losing the lift of the spine, lengthen up through the crown of your head. Try to balance your head over your pelvis. Make sure your shoulders are relaxed and are not riding up to your ears. Press your shoulder blades into your back. Lift your top chest and broaden your collarbones. Breathe fully. Open your body to receive the breath, remaining aware of how it feels to be in alignment. The benefits of mountain pose include the following:

- It teaches you how to stand correctly with proper alignment.
- It develops agility.
- It corrects minor misalignments of legs.
- It strengthens ankles.
- It relieves backache and neck strain.
- It opens the chest.

"A horse is the projection of peoples' dreams about themselves—strong, powerful, beautiful—and it has the capability of giving us escape from our mundane existence."

—Pam Brown

Go Horseback Riding

Just imagine bundling up in a sweater and scarf on a chilly spring or fall morning and riding a horse along a beach past crashing waves or through a leafy forest glade, replete with dew-laden spiderwebs and small critters scurrying out of your path. The world looks and feels different from the back of a horse. Horseback riding seems to heighten the senses of sight, smell, and touch. Riding at full gallop requires the use of those thigh muscles and feet and hands to stay in the saddle. Mounting and dismounting also can provide a little workout. But the joy of sitting atop a horse and observing the world awakening is a bonus for doing horseback riding as an exercise.

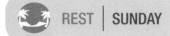

*"Yoga has a sly, clever way of short-circuiting the
mental patterns that cause anxiety."*

—Baxter Bell, quoted in *Yoga Journal*, March 2006

Practice Yoga to Relax

Specific yoga breathing techniques called *pranayama* are a great way
to relax at the end of a tough day. Pranayama both calm and strengthen
your respiratory and nervous systems, and when done correctly, have
many curative benefits, such as balancing and replenishing your body's
vital energy, lessening fatigue, and calming and quieting your mind and
emotions.

Conscious relaxation techniques used in yoga systematically guide
you into a state of deep relaxation. As the noisy chatter of your mind
recedes, your body is able to let go and release muscular tension. As
your body lets go, the breath rate slows and deepens, so the respiratory
system is allowed to rest. Slow, deep breathing encourages relaxation
and calmness just as a quick, shallow breath invites anxiety and action.

As your breath rate slows down, your heartbeat responds and also
becomes slower. This positively affects your entire circulatory system
and rests the heart, allowing it to rejuvenate. The sympathetic nervous
system, always ready to gear up for action, gets the message that it is
okay to relax, and then the parasympathetic nervous system initiates the
relaxation response.

The endocrine glands, responsible for much of your emotional and
physical well-being, receive the message to relax. (In this stress-driven
society, the adrenal glands in particular become overused and depleted.)

This deep relaxation goes to the very core of decreasing fatigue
and unraveling you from the inside out like a knotted ball of twine. You
emerge from this experience full of energy, as if you've just returned
from a mini-vacation from your stressful life.

"Legend has it that the Incan armies frequently marched for days at a time eating a mixture of quinoa and fat known as 'war balls,' and at planting time tradition demanded that the Incan leader would plant the first quinoa seed using a gold shovel."

—Jonny Bowden, PhD, CNS, author of *The 150 Healthiest Foods on Earth*

Try Quinoa Instead of Rice

Once known as "the gold of the Incas," this "grain-like" food—a complete protein—includes all nine essential amino acids, making it an excellent choice for vegetarians, vegans, and everyone else as well! Quinoa has extra-high amounts of the amino acid lysine, which is essential for tissue growth and repair. Combine this protein with quinoa's high amounts of potassium and its magnesium content to help lower your blood pressure and strengthen your heart. For such a small "grain," quinoa not only provides a whole lot of nutrients and helps boost your metabolism, but it may also be especially valuable for people with migraine headaches, diabetes, atherosclerosis, and other debilitating health issues. It is also a very good source of manganese as well as magnesium, iron, copper, phosphorus, and B vitamins—and it has a delicious nutty texture.

Tip: Soak and/or rinse raw quinoa to shed a bitter coating and reveal its nutty taste. Most boxed quinoa has already been soaked and/or rinsed and, like most boxed rices, will cook in approximately fifteen minutes.

WEEK THIRTY-FOUR

"Lack of activity destroys the good condition of every human being, while movement and methodical physical exercise save it and preserve it."

—Plato

Use a Medicine Ball to Play Catch

A great way to get a workout and have fun is to play catch with a partner using a medicine ball.

1. Standing firmly on your legs, hold the ball at the height of your chest.
2. Powerfully throw the ball straight out and away from you either at a partner who is ready to catch the ball or at a wall.
3. Have your hands out in front of you, ready to catch the ball as it returns to you. As you catch the ball, bring it in toward your chest to absorb the force in a gradual and fluid manner.
4. Repeat.

Another version of this exercise, which would be considered a progression, is to sit with your feet out in front of you. Place your feet hip width apart and bend your knees at about 90 degrees. Tilt your torso or upper body slightly back to engage your abdominal wall. Holding the ball at your chest, toss it to your partner (who can be sitting the same way) or against a wall. Catch the ball with your hands away from you and bring them in as you catch the ball.

*"Life is partly what we make it, and partly what
it is made by the friends we choose."*

—Tennessee Williams

Spend Time with Supportive Friends

A life rich with friends and loved ones can be one of the best elixirs when it comes to keeping our brains strong and vital. The importance of social support was demonstrated during a recent study at a large nursing home. Residents were randomly divided into three groups and given the task of completing a jigsaw puzzle. All were given four twenty-minute practice sessions, followed by a timed session. Members of the first group were given a lot of verbal encouragement by the experiment director during the practice sessions, members in the second group were given direct assistance, and members of the third group received neither encouragement nor assistance. Those in the group that received a lot of encouragement demonstrated marked improvement in both speed and proficiency in putting the puzzle together during the timed session. In other words, their mental acuity apparently improved. Those who were directly assisted did less well, and those who were left alone showed no change at all.

This demonstrates how social support in the form of interaction and encouragement can improve cognitive function in older people. However, it also demonstrates that the support must be appropriate to the individual and what he or she wishes to accomplish, whether it's a stronger memory or improved visual-spatial skills. Daily chats about the previous night's television shows may be seen as social support, but mere conversation with friends won't improve mental tasks. Invite your friends to join you in activities that involve something you'd like to master or learn more about, and then set aside at least one evening or afternoon when you can get together.

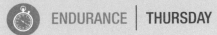

"My thoughts before a big race are usually pretty simple. I tell myself: Get out of the blocks, run your race, stay relaxed. If you run your race, you'll win. . . . Channel your energy. Focus."

—Carl Lewis, winner of nine Olympic gold medals

Add Bricks to Your Workouts

A brick is a bike ride followed by a run. One explanation for the term is that a brick is what your legs feel like after one of the workouts. No matter why it's called that, a brick can be a very effective triathlon training drill. For one thing, it simulates race day, when you will be starting the third phase of your triathlon, the run, immediately after racking up your bike. Bricks will train you to do something you probably have never done, as not many athletes would follow bike rides with runs without a reason. Plan to do a brick once a week.

1. There are two kinds of brick workouts, each emphasizing a different aspect of the training. In the first, you follow a ride of about seventy-five minutes with a run of fifteen minutes. Your ride will include some intervals—short periods of ramping up the pace followed by cool downs. The run will not be just a jog, but you will not push it.

2. Another brick workout consists of equal parts riding and running—forty-five minutes for each, for example—but the run is harder with interval workouts or at tempo pace (slightly faster than usual for the entire run).

No matter which brick workout you do, don't wait a long time before you start running. You should be running within five minutes of dismounting.

"Tree pose grows confidence."

—Terri Guillemets

Improve Balance and Coordination by Doing the Tree Pose

The tree pose (Vrksasana) develops balance and upward stretch, much like a tree, which has a strong, extensive root system, allowing it to grow tall and branch out. Start by standing in Tadasana (see Week Thirty-Three). Gaze straight ahead with a soft but focused gaze. Shift your weight to your left leg, root down, spread the balls of your feet, broaden your heels, and press firmly down with your big toe and little toe balls of your feet and the center of each heel. Turn your right foot out to the side. Then bring your right foot up to the inside of the left leg to where it is comfortable. You may use your hand to help bring the foot up the leg. Press the sole of the right foot against the inside of your left leg, leg against foot, as if they were pressing the spine up. If your foot does not easily stay on the leg, it is fine to leave it on the floor, turned out, with your right heel resting against the inner heel of your left foot. Maintain the grounding in your left foot and the extension in your left leg, taking care not to hyperextend the leg. Press the neck of your big toe down and lift your kneecap. Extend your arms out to the sides, with your palms facing up. Stretch all the way from the centerline in your body to your fingertips. On an inhalation, take the arms up over the head, stretching from your side ribs to your fingertips, palms facing each other. Continue breathing through your nostrils, relaxing your throat and diaphragm, and softening the front ribs and belly. Balance ease and effort. Stay in the tree pose for several breaths. To come out of the pose, exhale, and release your arms to the side as your right leg comes back into Tadasana. Repeat on the other side. The benefits of the tree pose include:

- It tones and strengthens legs muscles.
- It strengthens the ankles.
- It improves balance and coordination.
- It opens the hips.
- It lengthens the spine.
- It expands the chest for fuller breathing.

"Habitat gives us an opportunity which is very difficult to find: to reach out and work side by side with those who never have had a decent home—but work with them on a completely equal basis. It's not a big-shot, little-shot relationship. It's a sense of equality."

—former U.S. President Jimmy Carter

Volunteer with Habitat for Humanity

Swing a hammer, carry some lumber, and help build a home for a poor family, if this appeals to your social conscience. Habitat for Humanity (*www.habitat.org*) is a nonprofit organization that works in tandem with volunteers in communities worldwide to build houses for low-income people. Former President Jimmy Carter and his wife spend a week every year swinging hammers to help erect affordable shelter for the poor on behalf of Habitat for Humanity. To date, the organization has built more than 400,000 houses, sheltering more than two million people worldwide. If you believe that you could be doing more to help the less fortunate, then grab your hammer, get out there, and work up a sweat with—and for—people like yourself.

DON'T JUST RAISE A ROOF, RAISE AWARENESS

Another great way to help others is to raise awareness for the United Nation's World Habitat Day. Each year in October, events take place to focus on human settlement issues. Offer your support by counting down to it on your blog, posting it on your friends' Facebook walls, or sending an e-mail reminder to everyone in your address book. See *www.unhabitat.org* for more information.

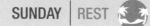

"It is not talking but walking that will bring us to heaven."

—Matthew Henry

Try a Walking Meditation

In Zen, walking meditation (kinhin) is the counterpart to sitting medita-tion (zazen), but walking meditation doesn't necessarily have anything to do with Zen. It is what it sounds like: meditation on the move. Walking meditation is different from sitting meditation because you have to be thinking about what you're doing so that you don't wander into traffic or bump into a tree. On the other hand, it isn't really so different, because in sitting meditation, you become acutely aware of your surroundings. They just aren't changing the way they change when you walk. Some people like to sit for most of their meditation session but then spend the last few minutes in walking meditation, and for some, who practice sitting meditation for longer periods of time, walking meditation gets the body moving periodically without breaking the meditative flow. To practice a walking meditation:

- Have a prepared path in mind so that you don't spend time think-ing about where to go during the meditation. Plot your path from beginning to end.
- Take time to breath slowly, centering yourself to prepare for the meditation.
- Take slow, deliberate steps. As you walk, notice how your breath feels as it comes in and out of your body. Notice how your limbs move, how your feet feel, how your hands and arms hang, the position of your torso, your neck, your head. Don't judge yourself as you walk. Just notice.
- Once you feel you've observed yourself well, begin to observe the environment around you as you walk. As soon as you catch your mind so wandering (and it will so wander), gently bring your thoughts back to your breathing.

243

"You can never have enough garlic. With enough garlic,
you can eat The New York Times.*"*

—Morley Safer

Pile on the Garlic

Garlic, one of the world's most popular culinary herbs, has a long history as a medicinal plant. Indeed, scientific studies have verified what herbalists have known for centuries—that garlic both prevents and treats illness in a wide variety of ways.

Among its many attributes, garlic is known to lower cholesterol levels, thin the blood, kill bacteria, boost the immune system, lower blood sugar levels, reduce the risk of certain types of cancer, and fire up the metabolic furnace. There is also evidence that the herb helps relieve asthma, eases ear infections, and facilitates healthy cell function. Bottom line: Those who wish to maintain their health and age well should eat lots of garlic.

Incorporate fresh garlic into salads by chopping, crushing, or putting it through a garlic press (two or three cloves a day is optimum). Whole garlic bulbs can be oven roasted and the individual cloves can be squeezed out onto bread or toast as a creamy spread.

WEEK THIRTY-FIVE

HOW TO ROAST GARLIC

Gather 4 cloves of garlic; ½ cup of chicken broth; 2 tablespoons of olive oil; ½ teaspoon of dried leaf thyme; ¼ teaspoon of ground black pepper; ¼ teaspoon of salt. Remove the outer peel from the garlic cloves and place each in a baking dish. Brush each clove with olive oil and then sprinkle with thyme, pepper and salt. Pour the chicken broth into the dish, cover the dish with foil, and bake at 350°F for 1 hour, basting frequently. Uncover the dish and bake at the same temperature for another 15 minutes.

"Strength training is not a contest. It's good for everybody."

—James Peterson, PhD, sports medicine consultant in Monterey, California

Add a High Knee Skip

Remember how much fun it was to skip as a child? Well, you can add this motion to your workout to strengthen your leg muscles and your overall strength and endurance. Here's how:

1. Swing the left knee up and simultaneously push off the right leg to jump off the floor.
2. The right arm swings forward as the left arm swings back.
3. Land with control on the right leg and step forward, moving right into the other side. Try to continuously alternate right and left with height being the goal rather than distance.

As your knee travels upward, push off the base leg and travel up. Although there is a slight amount of forward travel, the goal here is to go for height. Arm position can be a little tricky with this exercise.

Whatever knee travels upward, the opposite arm swings forward and up. This opposite arm swing is called a cross-extension pattern and is a very functional way to train because it is the pattern humans use to walk or move quickly. Again, be sure to control the landing and try to move from one rep to the next in a smooth and controlled manner.

> *"Ginkgo biloba powerfully enhances cerebral circulation, and has wondrous effects upon the brain."*
>
> —Dharma Singh Khalsa, MD, *Brain Longevity*

Take Ginkgo Biloba

The leaves of the ginkgo contain the active constituents ginkgo flavone glycosides and terpene lactones, the extract of which can be used to treat poor circulation in the legs as well as memory and cognitive problems. In a study published in the *Journal of the American Medical Association* researchers confirmed that people who take the ginkgo extract for mild to severe dementia may improve both their ability to remember and to interact socially. Usual dosage for extract: 120 to 240 milligrams daily, in three doses. Plan to take it for at least eight weeks before improvement shows. For capsules: Depending on capsule strength of the product you buy, use the same amount as the above recommended dosage. The standard dose is 40 to 60 milligrams. Buy a quality product and read the label. Look for products marked "24/6," an indication the product contains 24 percent flavone glycosides and 6 percent terpenes.

DON'T TAKE GINKGO IF . . .

Considered a brain-friendly herb, for reasons scientists don't understand, ginkgo may interfere with antidepressant MAO-inhibitor drugs such as phenelzine sulfate (Nardil) or tranylcypromine (Parnate). If you're on heart medication and want to take ginkgo, consult your doctor first. And be sure to stick to the recommended dosage of 120 to 240 milligrams a day.

"If you run 100 miles a week, you can eat anything you want—Why? Because (a) you'll burn all the calories you consume, (b) you deserve it, and (c) you'll be injured soon and back on a restricted diet anyway."

—Don Kardong

Cool Down with a Runner's Delight Smoothie

Any endurance runner feels amped before and pumped following a run. After all that hard work, you're definitely entitled to enjoy a sweet treat. Instead of undoing all that hard work with empty calories, indulge in the sweet taste of citrus with all its added benefits!

CITRUS SMOOTHIE

Recipe Yields: 3–4 cups

1 cup watercress
3 oranges, peeled
1 cup strawberries
1 cup raspberries
1 cup Greek-style yogurt

1. Combine watercress, oranges, berries, and ½ cup yogurt in a blender and blend until thoroughly combined.
2. Add remaining ½ cup yogurt as needed while blending until desired consistency is achieved.

PER 1 CUP SERVING: Calories 126 | **Fat** 0g | **Protein** 8g | **Sodium** 28mg | **Fiber** 6g | **Carbohydrates** 25g

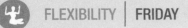

"Yoga is 99 percent practice and 1 percent theory."

—Sri Krishna Pattabhi Jois

Strengthen Your Ankles with the Eagle Pose

The eagle pose (Garudasan) entwines the arms and legs. Stand in Tadasana (see Week Thirty-Three). Extend your arms out to the sides. Bring them to the center and entwine your arms, crossing your left elbow over the inside of your right elbow. Turn your palms to face each other and join them. Lift your elbows to shoulder height and move your forearms away from your face to bring your wrists over your elbows. Bend your hips, knees, and ankles as if you are sitting. Cross your right leg over your left thigh. Press the toes and balls of your right foot down on the floor. On an exhalation, lift your right foot off the ground and wrap the right shin and foot around your left calf as best you can. Gaze straight ahead. Observe your breath coming into and expanding the space between your shoulder blades. Remain in the pose for several breaths and then return to Tadasana. Repeat on the other side.

If your balance is precarious, keep your foot on the floor. If your hands do not join, hold onto a strap with each hand. You can also practice with your back lightly against the wall for support.

As a variation, once you're in the pose, exhale and bend to the right for several breaths. Inhale and come back to center, and then exhale over to the left. Come back to center and then bend forward from the hips. Inhale and come back up into classic eagle pose.

The benefits of the eagle pose include the following:

- It improves circulation by squeezing and wringing out the arms and legs.
- It relieves shoulder stiffness.
- It strengthens the ankles.
- It helps reduce and prevent cramps in the calf muscles.

"A dog is one of the remaining reasons why some people can be persuaded to go for a walk."

—O. A. Battista

Take an Orphaned Dog for a Walk

Saturdays are a great day to take a long walk, so why not go to your local animal shelter and volunteer to take a dog for a walk? Then, if you find that enjoyable—and you likely will—why not sign up to volunteer regularly? In addition to walking dogs, you could do whatever needs to be done to help, even if it's something as simple as answering the phones. If dogs are your passion, consider joining other dog lovers to find homes for previously owned and rejected or abandoned animals. According to the Humane Society, animal shelters care for 6–8 million dogs and cats every year in the United States, of whom approximately 3–4 million are euthanized.

WALKING LOWERS YOUR RISK OF A HEART ATTACK

A study showed that older men who started walking about two miles a day had a 50 percent lower risk of heart attack than men who walked only a quarter mile. In addition, the study found that the risk of a heart attack dropped an additional 15 percent for every additional half mile walked per day.

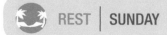

"Inhale, and God approaches you. Hold the inhalation, and God remains with you. Exhale, and you approach God. Hold the exhalation, and surrender to God."

—Krishnamacharya

Practice Yogic Breathing

The breath is the vehicle for *prana,* the vital life force. It is the universal energy that sustains all life. The prana enters the body upon inhalation, supplying every cell with energy, oxygen, and nutrients. With exhalation, waste and toxins are released. The breath is the bridge between the physical and spiritual worlds.

Yoga links the breath to the body. The breath is the bridge between mind and matter, between body and spirit. During inhalation, we are receiving life. Upon exhaling, we are returning what we don't need and ridding the body-mind of impurities. Inhalation is the movement of the self from the core to the periphery; exhalation is movement from the periphery to the core.

When you begin practicing yoga, your respiration may be shallow, with small, fairly rapid breaths. The average person breathes sixteen to eighteen breaths per minute. As you continue your yoga practice, your rate of breath will become slower, and each inhalation and exhalation will become longer and fuller. Deeper breaths allow the energy to reach every cell.

HAVING TROUBLE FALLING ASLEEP?

Try this technique developed by the Himalayan Institute. Pay attention to your breath, as you breathe through your nostrils. Gently slow down your exhalation until it's twice as long as the inhalation. Continue the two-to-one breathing ratio. Take eight breaths lying on your back, sixteen breaths lying on your right side, and thirty-two breaths lying on your left side.

"Fermented soy foods, like tempeh and miso, are a good source of iron. Soy foods are rich in copper and magnesium and are also rich in B vitamins. . . . Soybeans are rich in phytochemicals known as isoflavones, which may help prevent certain types of cancer, fight heart disease, and improve bone density."

—David W. Grotto, RD, LDN, *101 Foods That Could Save Your Life*

Try Some Tempeh

Tempeh is a fermented Indonesian protein substitute made from cultured grains or soy and a fungus starter called *Rhizopus oligosporus*. It is pressed into a block, packaged, and sold in health-food stores. Because it is the least processed among soy products, it is more digestible. Soy tempeh can be very low in carbohydrates, especially when you subtract the substantial amounts of fiber it provides. Tempeh is a complete protein food that contains all the essential amino acids. It is a very versatile food and a great vegetarian substitute for animal protein.

The fermentation process for tempeh also reduces levels of phytoestrogens and substances in soybeans that block thyroid function, mineral absorption, and glucose uptake in the brain. If homemade, tempeh can also be a valuable source of vitamin B_{12}.

WEEK THIRTY-SIX

YES, YOU CAN MAKE IT AT HOME!

It's easy to make tempeh at home at a very low cost. Dehulled soybeans are soaked overnight, cooked for about 30 minutes, and mixed with tempeh starter (available at health-food stores). After thirty-six to forty-eight hours incubation you have delicious fresh tempeh. Tempeh starter contains spores of *Rhizopus oligosporus* or *Rhizopus oryzae* which makes it vitamin B_{12} rich.

"I have always had good strength in my legs from working out with weights. I have also been riding a bike of some sort for most of my life and have good agility."

—Mark Paul Gosselaar

Add a Lateral Push to Your Workout

To add variety to your jumps, and to strengthen your leg muscles even farther, add lateral jumps to your workout. Lateral means to move away from the midline. So this exercise is done moving right to left in a continuous, smooth fashion. Begin by standing with most of your weight supported on your left leg. Wait until you have stabilized your weight on your left leg, and then begin extending your right leg outward. As your right foot moves to your right, push off with your left leg to cover as much distance as you can. You want to land softly and firmly on your right leg, with the ability to push off again in the opposite direction. Remember to absorb the landing by bending at your hips and knees. Keep moving from side to side, each time doing so with a bend and push from your supporting leg. You may find that a slight swing of your arms is helpful in developing a little more power. Your arms will also help stabilize your landing.

Go slowly until you have the ability to land squarely on each foot, with knees slightly bent. As your skill improves, you can add continuous motion and a fluid leap from one leg to the other to heighten the exercise. However, the lateral push is not meant to develop your speed. So going faster than is necessary or safe is not going to help you improve. Take your time so that you can really develop a nice strong pushoff that can cover an acceptable and challenging distance.

"When I do get time, I like to hike and I take lots of vitamins and powders to keep healthy."

—Catherine Bell

Make Magnesium a Priority

This mineral is an absolute must for proper brain function in that it aids neuron metabolism, helps reduce brain damage from ischemia (a lack of blood flow to the brain), and boosts the effectiveness of certain antioxidants. Magnesium may also play a role in the prevention of Alzheimer's disease, since studies show that the brains of most AD patients are magnesium-deficient, but excessively high in calcium. (In healthy brains, the two minerals have a relatively equal ratio.) Every cell in the body needs magnesium. Magnesium is a requirement for more than 300 body enzymes, body chemicals that regulate all kinds of body functions. This mineral helps maintain normal nerve and muscle function, keeps heart rhythm steady, and helps keep bones strong. Deficiency can result from an increase in urine output—like that caused by diuretics—poorly controlled diabetes, and alcoholism. The UL (Tolerable Upper Intake Level) for magnesium is 350 mg per day for adults over eighteen, and too much is not harmful unless the mineral is not excreted properly due to disorders such as kidney disease.

Choose Foods Rich in Magnesium

Magnesium can be found in a wide variety of foods. The best sources include legumes, almonds, avocados, toasted wheat germ, wheat bran, fish, seafood, fruits, fruit juice, pumpkin seeds, and whole grains. Green vegetables, especially cooked spinach, can be good sources too.

"Through my illness I learned rejection. I was written off.
That was the moment I thought, Okay, game on.
No prisoners. Everybody's going down."

—Lance Armstrong

Join a Cycling Club

Cycling is a great way to build endurance, but why not have fun while pedaling your way to health? Plus, there's safety in numbers, particularly when you are cycling along a roadway. Our best advice: Do your bicycle training in group rides as often as possible. Besides being more enjoyable because of the social aspect, a group ride is safer. For example, a group of fifteen to twenty cyclists is easier for drivers to see than one or two on their own. Besides, your fellow riders are likely to push you harder to keep up with them, to encourage you when you think you're too tired to go one more mile, and to inspire you to greater heights. When it comes to cycle training, cycling outdoors with friends is a great way to stay motivated—and to have fun.

A FEW TIPS

When selecting a course for your cycling workouts, safety is the number one concern. Consult your local bicycle shop for information on riding courses. The bike shop owners will know several, and they will probably have some organized rides you can take part in as well.

When searching on your own, look for wide roads without heavy traffic. In many areas, roads and city streets have bike lanes. At the very least, look for wide roads with good-sized shoulders or breakdown lanes. Avoid two-lane roads with no shoulders.

*"The last time I opened my chakra so I could feel my peace,
I got thrown right out of the pub."*

—Terri Guillemets

Revitalize and Relax by Inverting Your Legs

To do the legs-up-the-wall pose (Viparita Karani) place a bolster or one to three horizontally folded blankets against a wall. Lie on your side with your left hip on the support, buttocks close to the wall, and your knees bent. Roll onto your back and swing your legs up the wall. Your legs should be resting against the wall, your lower back and sacrum on the support, and the rest of your torso flat on the floor. Stretch your arms out horizontally, with your palms facing up. Your eyes may close and soften. Breathe naturally and enjoy the relaxation and revitalization of the pose. To come out of the pose, bend your knees and roll over onto your right side. Using your hands, press yourself up to a seated position. You can also practice Viparita Karani with your legs separated wide apart. Or you can bend your knees slightly if it is too intense a stretch for the hamstring muscles. The benefits of legs up the wall pose include the following:

- It drains fluid from the legs.
- It softens the belly and groin.
- It reverses the effects of gravity.
- It reverses the flow of blood and lymph.
- It rests the heart and the brain.
- It relieves tired legs.
- It revitalizes and relaxes.

"I never saw a discontented tree. They grip the ground as though they liked it, and though fast rooted they travel about as far as we do. They go wandering forth in all directions with every wind, going and coming like ourselves, traveling with us around the sun two million miles a day, and through space heaven knows how fast and far!"

—John Muir

Plant a Tree

What better way to enjoy a day than to spend one planting a tree? Trees are not only beautiful, they absorb carbon dioxide and release oxygen into the atmosphere. As such, all urban areas can benefit from having more trees. One tree gives enough oxygen back through photosynthesis to support two human beings. To discover other interesting facts about trees, go to *www.coloradotrees.org/benefits*.

If you don't have space on your property for a new tree, call your city government to see if they'd welcome one in the park or other common areas. Offer to plant the tree in honor of a citizen who has served the city or the country well, such as town founders, mayors, or anyone who died while in the armed forces.

TAKE A FLIGHT, PLANT A TREE

It can be hard to avoid taking flights, especially if you need to get from one side of the world to another. However, those long flights have a negative impact on our environment. Luckily, there is a way you can offset the damage caused by the fuel used. Treeflights will plant trees to help offset the damage caused to the environment by your flight (*www.treeflights.com*).

"Stillness and action are relative, not absolute, principles. It is important to find a balance of yin and yang, not just in Qigong, but in everyday life. In movement, seek stillness and rest. In rest, be mindful and attentive."

—Ken Cohen, *The Way of Qigong: The Art and Science of Chinese Energy Healing*

Try Qigong

Qigong is an ancient Chinese Taoist martial arts form dating back at least 2,500 years. (Some Chinese archeologists have found references to Qigong-like techniques at least 5,000 years old.) Like its successor, Tai Chi, Qigong involves specific, fluid, dance-like movements and postures, as well as massage, meditation, and gentle breathing to maintain and improve overall health and balance the body's internal energy (called *chi* in China).

While it's considered a supplementary form of healing, Qigong has been shown to improve posture and respiration, induce the relaxation response, cause favorable changes in blood chemistry, and improve self-awareness and concentration. Research suggests that Qigong may be beneficial for asthma, arthritis, cancer, cardiovascular disease, chronic fatigue, fibromyalgia, headaches, pain, and a wide variety of common ailments.

"It's bizarre that the produce manager is more important to my children's health than the pediatrician."

—Meryl Streep

Eat Kale and Other Brassica Vegetables

Loaded with cancer-fighting antioxidants, kale is, literally, one of the healthiest foods in the vegetable kingdom. Together with its cousin, broccoli, kale offers strong protection against cancer and other disease. Kale and other Brassica vegetables contain a potent glucosinolate phytonutrient, which actually boosts your body's detoxification enzymes, clearing potentially carcinogenic substances more quickly from your body. More common members of the prestigious Brassica family of vegetables include: cabbage, broccoli, brussels sprouts, cauliflower, kale, collards, mustard greens, rapini, bok choy, and broccoli rabe. With so many choices take advantage of having one variety each day of the week.

"Muscles come and go; flab lasts."

—Bill Vaughan

Bolster Your Body's Health with Vitamin C

Eating a balanced diet of vibrant fruits, vegetables, and leafy greens can ensure you're providing for your health and your athletic ability.

VIVACIOUS VITAMIN C

Recipe Yields: 3–4 cups
1 cup watercress
½ pineapple, peeled and cored
3 oranges, peeled
1 lemon, peeled
1 cup strawberries
1 cup purified water

1. Combine watercress, pineapple, oranges, lemon, strawberries, and ½ cup water in a blender and blend until thoroughly combined.
2. Add remaining ½ cup water as needed while blending until desired consistency is achieved.

PER 1 CUP SERVING | **Calories** 138 | **Fat** 0g | **Protein** 3g | **Sodium** 7mg | **Fiber** 4g | **Carbohydrates** 35g

---

VITAMINS AND MINERALS FOR PROACTIVE HEALTH

How important is vitamin C to an athlete? When was the last time you saw a top-performing athlete take first place hacking and heaving all the way to the finish line? Never! If you're going to keep your body in top shape, ready for anything, sound nutrition isn't the only thing requiring attention. In order to get the biggest bang for your buck out of performance nutrition, load up on vibrant fruits and veggies that do double duty.

"To all my little Hulkamaniacs, say your prayers,
take your vitamins, and you will never go wrong."

—Hulk Hogan

Keep Potassium Levels High

Potassium is an electrolyte that works closely with its counterparts, chloride and sodium. Over 95 percent of potassium is in the body's cells and helps regulate the flow of fluids and minerals in and out of the body's cells. It also helps maintain normal blood pressure, maintain heart and kidney function, and transmit nerve impulses and contraction of muscles. Studies have also shown that potassium may also reduce the risk of high blood pressure and stroke. Potassium is very important in converting blood sugar into glycogen, the storage form of blood sugar in your muscles and liver. Potassium is widely available in foods, but chronic diarrhea, vomiting, diabetic acidosis, kidney disease, or prolonged use of laxatives or diuretics could cause a deficiency. Most people excrete excess potassium in their urine. If the excess cannot be excreted—for instance, in the case of someone with kidney disease—it can cause heart problems. Some experts recommend a higher intake, around 3,500 milligrams per day, to help protect against high blood pressure.

CHOOSE FOODS RICH IN POTASSIUM

A diet low in fat and cholesterol and rich in foods containing potassium, magnesium, and calcium—such as fruits, vegetables, legumes, and dairy foods—has shown evidence of reducing blood pressure. Potassium-rich foods include fresh meat, poultry, fish, figs, lentils, kidney beans, black beans, baked potatoes (with skin), avocados, orange juice, cantaloupes, bananas, and cooked spinach.

"The man who is swimming against the
stream knows the strength of it."

—Woodrow T. Wilson

Strengthen Your Leg Muscles via Deep Water Running

A great cross-training activity is deep water running. In deep water running, you are suspended vertically in a pool by wearing a flotation belt around your waist or torso. Although your feet don't touch the bottom of the pool, you then simulate running.

This cross-training activity is just what the doctor ordered for the rehabilitation of injuries or overuse of leg muscles. Additionally, because there is no shock from footstrike, deep water running is a perfect alternative to a midweek easy day run or power walk. The resistance of the water gives you all the benefits of running or power walking but none of the stress or shock of footstrike associated with power walking or road running. Even though it is possible to run in the water without floatation aids, find a pool that offers these devices (such as vests or belts) for a workout at once easier on your upper body yet more specific in targeting your leg muscles.

WHY RUNNING IS SO HARD ON YOUR BODY

It is estimated that every step you take as you run makes an impact on your body equal to up to six times your body weight. This puts stress on the bones and joints, especially when just starting out. Swimming and cycling are low-impact activities; running is a high-impact sport.

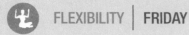

*"Yoga teaches us to cure what need not be endured
and endure what cannot be cured."*

—B.K.S. Iyengar

Add Downward Facing Dog to Your Practice

If you've ever seen a dog stretching, you know that this pose looks like an upside down V. Start on your hands and knees. Place your hands under your shoulders and your knees directly under your hips. Your inner arms face each other and your elbows are straight and firm. Let your shoulder blades come onto your back. Observe that your upper arm bones connect into the shoulder socket. Your pelvis is in a neutral position, horizontal to the floor. Tuck your toes under. Plant your hands firmly on the floor and spread your fingers evenly apart. Press your palms, knuckles, and fingers into the floor. Your hands are part of the pose's foundation, and they must stay rooted in order for extension of the spine to occur. Inhale, lift your hips evenly, and press your hands and feet down. On the exhalation, straighten your legs and let your head drop between your arms. Press the front of your thighs back to elongate your torso. Press your hands down, extending into your fingertips. Then stretch your arms away from your hands, all the way up to your buttock bones. Let your spine lengthen from the top of your head to your tailbone, into one long line of extension. Lift your heels up, and continue stretching all the way up the back of your legs to your buttock bones. Now lengthen your heels down, but keep stretching the back of your legs up. Lift your kneecaps and firm your thighs. Your heels are stretching toward the floor. Lift your shins out of the top of your ankles as you press your heels down. Your feet are also working, spreading, grounding, with arches lifting to enhance the upward extension of your legs. Fully stretch your legs. Keep your arms as long as possible. Bending your elbows will make it difficult to transfer the weight of your body from your arms to your legs. Remain in the pose for several breaths, extending your spine on the inhalation. Then bend your knees and come down.

"It is by riding a bicycle that you learn the contours of a country best, since you have to sweat up the hills and coast down them. Thus you remember them as they actually are, while in a motor car only a high hill impresses you, and you have no such accurate remembrance of country you have driven through as you gain by riding a bicycle."

—Ernest Hemingway

Take a Biking Vacation

Like walking trips, biking trips can range from the flat-terrained, gentle journeys from elegant inn to elegant inn, to the more strenuous hilly tours carrying a tent on your bicycle.

One good thing about bicycle trips is that you can cover a lot of ground (or at least more than you do when you walk) on your trip and, usually, you decide how much you ride each day. Most trip organizers have a van to carry luggage, food, and other necessities, so you can ride unencumbered and, if you get tired, they'll give you a lift in that van.

The organizers of biking trips will also help you determine what level trip you should join. Serious cyclists will want to cover longer distances and will look for hills to climb, while the more leisurely cyclist should choose trips that are on flat ground or that offer some walking (the van will carry your bike) as well as riding.

"Massage is an excellent stress management tool. It helps your body and mind to relax as it encourages the body to help heal itself."

—Melissa Roberts, theologian and stress management specialist

Try Shiatsu and Acupressure

Shiatsu is the Japanese word for finger pressure and is sometimes known as acupressure. Shiatsu is an ancient form of massage, still widely practiced, that involves the application of pressure through fingers, palms, elbows, or knees to pressure points in the body. Pressure points are certain points along energy meridians that the Japanese and other Asian cultures have defined within the body. Pressure on these points is thought to release energy blockages that cause pain and disease, resulting in balance, equilibrium, and greater physical health. Acupuncture is based on the same principle but uses very thin needles painlessly inserted into pressure points. Although the idea may sound strange to a Westerner, much research has supported the effectiveness of both acupuncture and acupressure in the relief of pain and the treatment of certain disorders.

"You know, when you get your first asparagus, or your first acorn squash, or your first really good tomato of the season, those are the moments that define the cook's year. I get more excited by that than anything else."

—Mario Batali

Have Fresh Asparagus for Dinner

Asparagus provides tons of folic acid, potassium, and fiber, and is a heart-healthy source of vitamins A, C, and K. It also contains the carbohydrate inulin, which promotes the growth and activity of good bacteria in your intestines—and it's a diuretic.

TOFU AND ASPARAGUS STIR-FRY

Serves 6

½ tablespoon peanut oil
1 teaspoon sesame oil
1 cup vegetable broth
2 cups fresh asparagus, cut in 2-inch segments
1 16-ounce package firm tofu, cubed
1 clove fresh garlic, minced
½ teaspoon all-purpose seasoning
1 cup green onions, sliced
1 tablespoon ground ginger
1 tablespoon low-sodium soy sauce
1 tablespoon Worcestershire
1 teaspoon Splenda brown sugar
1 teaspoon cornstarch
2 tablespoons sesame seeds

1. Coat a large skillet with nonstick spray and heat over medium heat. Add peanut oil, sesame oil, vegetable broth, and asparagus. Cook for 8 to 10 minutes.
2. Add remaining ingredients to skillet. Stirring often, cook for 15 to 20 minutes or until asparagus are tender and sauce thickens.

"Now for the big bang! Power training is very explosive at its highest levels. Plyometrics are a great way to develop muscular power."

—Jeff Levine, Krav Maga instructor

Add Plyometric Exercises to Bolster Your Workout

Plyometrics are resistance exercises that use your own body weight as the resistance. Not only are they convenient, plyometrics are effective for body control because they build explosive power, strength, balance, and coordination. In terms of everyday fitness, plyometric conditioning is the most useful and appropriate type of training. When added into a workout that includes cardio conditioning, you have a complete regimen. Because plyometrics don't require any equipment, they involve no extra cost and can be done in a relatively small space, which means they are useful exercises for those who travel, work out at the office, or for anyone who gets the sudden urge to work on conditioning.

Plyometric exercises include pushups (performed so explosively that your body and hands leave the ground), jumping squats, jumping lunges, and throwing a medicine ball forward, up, or explosively in any direction. With all plyometrics, you will need to start slowly and build up speed as your strength grows. We have specifics for plyometric pushups, jumping squats, jumping lunges, and lateral pushes coming up. Meanwhile, see if you can come up with other ideas for ways you can use your body weight to bolster your workout.

"Get off your horse and drink your milk."

—John Wayne

Consider Calcium Supplements

Calcium's primary function is to help build and maintain bones and teeth. In addition, calcium helps blood clot, helps your muscles contract and your heartbeat, helps regulate blood pressure, plays a role in normal nerve function and nerve transmission, and helps regulate the secretion of hormones and digestive enzymes. In a review of twenty-two studies, calcium supplementation was found to moderately reduce blood pressure in adults with hypertension, or high blood pressure, but had little effect on people with normal blood pressure.

Calcium has a UL set at 2,500 mg per day for adults and children. When consuming supplements up to this amount, no adverse effects are likely. However, higher doses over an extended period of time may cause kidney stones and poor kidney function as well as reduce the absorption of other minerals such as iron and zinc. Consult with your doctor before adding supplements.

CHOOSE FOODS RICH IN CALCIUM

Some of the best sources of calcium are foods in the dairy group, such as milk, cheese, and yogurt. In addition, some dark green leafy vegetables, such as broccoli, spinach, kale, and collards, are good sources. Other good sources include fish with edible bones, such as sardines and salmon, as well as calcium-fortified soymilk, tofu made with calcium, shelled almonds, cooked dried beans, calcium-fortified cereals, and calcium-fortified orange juice.

"I always wanted to be Peter Pan, the boy who never grows up. I can't fly, but swimming is the next best thing. It's harmony and balance. The water is my sky."

—Clayton Jones

Do Jumping Jacks in a Pool

Pool workouts are a great way to warm up, but also to strengthen muscles. Jumping jacks done in water strengthen your gluteals, adductors, and abductors (hips, buttocks, inner thighs, outer thighs). Here's how to do them:

1. Stand in chest-deep water with your feet close together. Bend your knees slightly, lengthen your spine, relax your shoulders.
2. Perform a jumping jack movement. If you are toning the outer thighs, focus on powering out as you jump, returning gently to center. If you are toning the inner thighs, focus on powering in as you jump, returning gently to a wide stance.
3. Inhale to prepare, exhale on the power phase. Inhale on the return phase. Keep tone in your abdominals. Maintain good posture with neutral spinal alignment. Avoid arching your back. Land softly and with control. Use arms to assist your balance.

Variations to increase the challenge:

- Increase size of movement on the power phase.
- Increase speed of movement on the power phase.
- Increase height of jumps.
- Perform exercise in shallower water.
- Use an aquatic step. Start with both legs on the pool floor behind step. Perform jacks with power phase. Jump up on step. If you are toning the outer thighs, focus on powering out as you jump down and straddle the step. If you are toning the inner thighs, focus on powering in as you jump up onto the step. Using the aquatic step is the most difficult level since the force of gravity is increased.

"Yoga is the fountain of youth. You're only as young as your spine is flexible."

—Bob Harper

Add Variations of the Cat-Cow Pose

Begin in basic cat-cow pose (see Week Twenty-Eight). Inhale and lengthen your spine. Exhale and draw your right knee and your chin into your chest while rounding your back. Repeat this pattern five times and then change sides. You can also try starting on all fours and shifting your weight onto your right hip. Inhale and lengthen your spine. Exhale and turn your head to look at your right hip. With each successive exhalation, try to bring your head closer to the hip. This action will create stretch on the left side of your body and contraction on the right side of your body. As you inhale, feel the breath come into your left side, which has been stretched and opened to receive the breath. Once you've gone as far as you can go (without aggressive action), come back to center, and then repeat on the left side. The cat-cow pose and its variations have the following benefits:

- They increase the flexibility and suppleness of the spine and its surrounding muscles.
- They work the entire spine.
- They stretch and tone the muscles of the back.
- They plump up the spinal discs and aid in fluid circulation in and out of the discs.
- They stimulate the nervous system.
- They're useful as a warm-up for other postures and as a way of stretching the backside of the body after back bending.
- They teach coordination of the breath with movement.
- They release tension in the back.

*"There can be no greater issue than that of
conservation in this country."*

—Theodore Roosevelt

Become a Conservation Volunteer

A great way to get exercise, learn about ecology, botany, local wildlife, and public land management issues, and make a valuable contribution to your local community is to work with local parks and recreation departments to restore natural habitats. Tasks might include constructing a path, clearing a hiking trail, dry stone walling, planting some trees and bushes, or whatever needs to be done to preserve or create green spaces in your community.

Another way to help is to make a donation to The Corps Network, an organization that carries on the tradition of America's Civilian Conservation Corps in restoring the environment. For information on the organization and to learn how to donate, see *www.nascc.org*.

CIVILIAN ROOTS

The Civilian Conservation Corps (CCC) was a public work relief program created by President Franklin D. Roosevelt as part of the New Deal. It provided work for young men whose families were unable to find jobs during the Great Depression. During the time it operated, between 1933 and 1942, CCC volunteers planted nearly 3 billion trees to help reforest America, constructed more than 800 parks nationwide, upgraded most state parks, updated forest fire fighting methods, and built a network of service buildings and public roadways in remote areas.

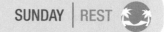

"Yoga means union—the union of body with consciousness and consciousness with the soul. Yoga cultivates the ways of maintaining a balanced attitude in day-to-day life and endows skill in the performance of one's actions."

—B.K.S. Iyengar

Adopt the Practice of Yoga to Renew Your Spirit

Yoga is one of the oldest *holistic* health-care systems in existence, focusing on both the mind and the body. In the Western world, most people live in their heads more than in their bodies. The educational system is focused on book learning; many jobs are either cerebral or mindless (few incorporate both). And yet Western medicine focuses almost solely on the physical aspect of health, neglecting the emotional and spiritual aspects that yoga attends to.

Through the practice of yoga postures and breath work, you can reconnect your body and mind and discover your spirit. You can become whole and regain an intimate knowledge of your real Self (not the little self with needs and wants that gnaws at you all day long). Yoga is the art of listening to all parts of your Self.

This ancient practice is a spiritual discipline with a code of ethics toward yourself and others. It is not a religion. It is a system for discovering and developing the true Self, an ancient method of psychotherapy (before there was one), and a potent self-evolutionary tool. In the classic text the *Yoga Sutras,* the spiritual path of yoga is laid out like a roadmap with discussion of the mental, physical, and psychological benefits and roadblocks along the way.

*"Because you don't live near a bakery doesn't mean
you have to go without cheesecake."*

—Hedy Lamarr

Make It a Cheesecake Night

Yes, you can (occasionally) have your cheesecake and eat it too! Here's a basic fat-free cheesecake recipe that you can build on by sampling various flavors of extracts and adding unique ingredients like graham cracker bits, pretzel pieces, fruit, and small bits of dark chocolate.

FITZ'S LOW-FAT CHEESECAKE

Serves 8
3 8-ounce packages fat-free cream cheese, softened
¾ cup Splenda
1 teaspoon vanilla extract
¾ cup Egg Beaters
1 prepared low-fat graham cracker crust

1. In an electric mixer, combine cream cheese, Splenda, and vanilla on medium speed. Add Egg Beaters and mix until well blended. Pour mixture into crust.
2. Bake at 350°F for 40 minutes or until center is almost set. Cool and refrigerate for 2 hours or overnight.

PER SERVING: Calories 240 | **Fat** 9g | **Protein** 15g | **Sodium** 666mg | **Fiber** 0g | **Carbohydrates** 29g

"The higher your energy level, the more efficient your body. The more efficient your body, the better you feel and the more you will use your talent to produce outstanding results."

—Anthony Robbins

Add Plyometric Pushups to Your Daily Workout

There are a few variations of plyometric (using your body weight as resistance, see Week Thirty-Eight) pushups. Whatever variation you choose, the concept is the same. The first time you perform this exercise keep your knees on the floor. Once you have built some power in the upper body you may progress to doing the exercise on your toes. Keep in mind that it is much more challenging for women to do these exercises on their toes. Be smart about your progressions. Many elite female athletes only do these exercises with their knees on the floor.

1. Place your hands the same way you would for a pushup.
2. Move to the bottom of your pushup.
3. Similar to a squat jump, push down with your hands in order to go up.
4. Push with enough force that your hands leave the floor.
5. Clap your hands together (or attempt to do so).
6. Land softly by bending your elbows to bring your chest toward the floor.
7. Prepare for the next rep.

Continue moving down and up with controlled landings on the arms.

You can also perform this exercise by pushing off the ground and touching your shoulders upon takeoff. Another version is clapping the hands behind the back. One of the most advanced versions is with one hand elevated on a ball and switching hands while in the air. This version is challenging because not only do you have to get more height, but your body has to move in space to switch sides.

"A Jewish woman had two chickens. One got sick, so the woman made chicken soup out of the other one to help the sick one get well."

—Henny Youngman

Protect Your Brain Cells with Selenium

This very powerful antioxidant benefits the brain by preventing oxidation of fat. Why is this important? It's important because more than half of the brain is composed of a type of fat. By inhibiting oxidation, selenium slows age-related brain deterioration and preserves cognitive function. Selenium also benefits the immune system, and some studies suggest that it improves circulation throughout the body. Because selenium levels tend to decline with age, older people should take selenium supplements in addition to adding selenium-rich foods to their diets.

Selenium also works with glutathione peroxidase to keep potentially damaging free radicals under control. In Japan, where people traditionally consume about 500 micrograms of selenium a day, the cancer rate is nearly five times lower than in countries where daily selenium intake is less.

Don't Overdo Selenium

There is no established RDA for selenium, though men and women can safely consume between 50 and 200 micrograms daily, not exceeding 400 mcg per day for adults over eighteen. It's important not to overdo selenium, as it can become toxic if 700 micrograms are consumed on a daily basis.

CHOOSE FOODS RICH IN SELENIUM

Natural sources of selenium include broccoli, cabbage, celery, cucumbers, garlic, onions, kidney, liver, chicken, whole-grain foods, seafood, and milk.

"Nothing in the world is more flexible and yielding than water. Yet when it attacks the firm and the strong, none can withstand it, because they have no way to change it. So the flexible overcome the adamant, the yielding overcome the forceful. Everyone knows this, but no one can do it."

—Lao Tzu

Take Swimming Classes or Hire a Swimming Coach

Few people instinctively know the right way to swim. In that sport, technique is everything. The best way to get better as a swimmer is by enlisting the aid of a coach. A coach often works with a group, watching each swimmer in turn and offering tips for better technique and form. Fortunately, most facilities with big pools also have programs that include coaches as part of their master swim classes.

Those who consider themselves athletically prepared to participate in triathlons are able to swim 500 to 1,000 yards in relative comfort without extended breaks. Think you're at that level? Think again. Swimming pools where athletes train are basically the same size, and most are 25 yards long. A mile is 1,760 yards, so to do a 1-mile swim you would have to swim from one end of the pool to the other and back again thirty-five times.

Add swimming to your workouts and slowly increase the number of laps you can do, aiming for quantity over speed. To build endurance, the longer you swim is more important than how fast you do the laps. In the pool, your goal is to achieve long, smooth strokes that carry you a greater distance. Hit the pool a few days a week, even if it's just for short workouts, say twenty or thirty minutes at a time.

GOOD NEWS!

Swimming programs are not terribly expensive, usually $25 to $30 per month, and the costs include a coach. A typical masters swim program usually provides buoys, kickboards, and other equipment you can use to bolster your workouts.

"You cannot do yoga. Yoga is your natural state. What you can do are yoga exercises, which may reveal to you where you are resisting your natural state."

—Sharon Gannon

Go from Cat-Cow Pose to Threading the Needle

Begin in basic cat-cow pose (see Week Twenty-Eight). Starting on all fours, thread your right arm under your body to the left side. Rest your right ear and the top of your right shoulder on the floor. Your left arm is bent at a 90-degree angle and the palm is flat on the floor. Take several breaths in this position. If comfortable, place your left palm on the *sacrum* (the small of the back). This will increase the intensity of the pose somewhat, so go back if the first position is enough for you. With each exhalation, draw your left shoulder and elbow easily behind you. Stay for several breaths and then unthread your right arm and come back to cat-cow position. Take a slow breath, and then repeat the same pose by threading your left arm under your body. The cat-cow pose and its variations increase the flexibility and suppleness of your spine and its surrounding muscles, because they stretch and tone the muscles and stimulate your nervous system, improving circulation.

*"I've learned that making a 'living' is not the
same thing as 'making a life.'"*

—Maya Angelou

Take an Adventure Vacation

For bold travelers, there's nothing more exciting than an adventure vacation. Not only do you get to experience a place you've never seen before, but you also get to challenge yourself physically and keep in shape. This type of vacation can go in many directions. Are you interested in biking? Perhaps you'd like to bike through France, stopping at hostels along the way. Do you like running in races? Why not follow a trail of 5K races all over New England in the spring? Here are some other ideas that might fulfill your adventurous whims.

- Walk the outback of Australia.
- Learn to surf in Hawaii.
- Learn to sail in the British Virgin Islands.
- Bicycle through Baja California.
- Hike to Machu Picchu.
- Helihike in British Columbia.

The important thing to remember about these trips is that they require training. Even if you're very active, you need to train specifically for the type of trip you're going to take. Ask the group you're going with to advise you on ways you can get in shape to get the most out of your trip.

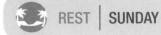

"Happiness is not a matter of intensity but of balance, order, rhythm, and harmony."

—Thomas Merton

Identify Precisely What Is Causing Your Stress

Often, when you feel "stressed out," it is a generalized feeling of stress. If you take a moment to examine your situation, however, you will find that your feelings are actually the cumulative result of numerous individual pressures that have finally reached the boiling point. One of the first steps toward learning how to manage stress effectively is to identify these individual pressures—the types of things in your life that cause you stress. Your awareness is the first step. The next time you start to feel overwhelmed and stressed out, explore these feelings in greater depth. Ask yourself the following questions to determine what is causing these emotions:

- Am I overcommitted?
- Am I taking care of others and neglecting my own self-care?
- Am I trying to accomplish everything on my own without asking for any support from anyone else?
- Are my expectations unrealistic?
- What is going on in my life right now that gives me a sense of struggle?
- Is what I stress over more important than my health and happiness?

If you are the type of person who finds it helpful to keep a journal, try to record things that trigger your stress. Write down what happened, what you were thinking or feeling, and how you reacted physically. This can give you valuable insight into the cumulative triggers you face throughout the day. Then consider the importance of those things and the importance of your long-term health and well-being. Consider the effects of stress on your health and mood and how that then affects those around you. Is what you stress over more concerning than premature death and disability? If not, then it is worth learning how to manage your stress.

"Every superfood is going to be a 'real' (unprocessed) food . . .
You don't find fortified potato chips in the superfood category."

—Elizabeth Somer, *The Essential Guide to Vitamins and Minerals*

Boost Your Vitamin Consumption with Sea Vegetables

Gram for gram, sea vegetables—seaweeds and algae—are higher in essential vitamins and minerals than any other known food group. These minerals are bio-available to the body in chelated, colloidal forms that make them more easily absorbed. Sea vegetables that provide minerals in this colloidal form have been shown to retain their molecular identity while remaining in liquid suspension. The following is a descriptive list of what sea vegetables can add to your daily diet:

- They can contain as much as 48 percent protein.
- They are a rich source of both soluble and insoluble dietary fiber.
- The brown sea varieties—kelp, wakame, and kombu—contain alginic acid, which has been shown to remove heavy metals and radioactive isotopes from the digestive tract.
- They contain significant amounts of vitamin A, in the form of beta-carotene, as well as vitamins B, C, and E.
- They are high in potassium, calcium, sodium, iron, and chloride.
- They provide the fifty-six minerals and trace minerals that your body requires to function properly.

Today sea vegetables are available from the Maine Coast Sea Vegetable Company on the east coast and the Mendocino Sea Vegetable Company in northern California. Add them to green smoothies for a nutritional punch.

WEEK FORTY

"Once stability and strength has been established and achieved it is then safe to add power training through plyometric exercises to your training program."

—Tina Angelotti, developer of the Krav Maga fitness program

Add Plyometric Squat Jumps

Vertical jumps are an advanced variation of a squatting exercise, and exercises that involve leaving the ground are a great way to develop power—if your core is solid and you can withstand the impact.

1. With your feet about shoulder width apart, sit your hips back and down while keeping your back straight, as if you were about to sit down in a chair, bending your knees in a squat.
2. Place your arms down and back behind you.
3. From the bottom of your squat, swing your arms overhead and push down with your legs, moving your hips forward and up in order to jump off the ground.
4. After leaving the ground you must land appropriately. Use your hips and knees to absorb the landing. You should land back on the ground with a fluid and light movement. The landing should not feel jarring at all. Your arms should swing back upon landing and upward upon the take off. Try to find a smooth rhythm of legwork and arm swing so that one jump leads into the next in a continuous manner.

The faster you are able to generate large forces moving down into the floor, the higher and more powerful your jump will be. Once you are comfortable with this movement you can emphasize jumping higher, or swinging the arms faster, in order to produce more power by using the momentum of the arm swing. The same jump can be performed without using any arm swing at all. Place your hands on your hips and observe the difference in the height of your jump. Without the arm swing this becomes much more challenging.

"There's no such thing as soy milk. It's soy juice."

—Lewis Black

Protect Your DNA with Zinc

This mineral aids the brain as part of a metabolic process that eliminates harmful free radicals. It also strengthens neuronal membranes for greater protection and helps get rid of lead, which can enter the brain through automobile exhaust and other sources and adversely affect mental function. Zinc is part of the molecular structure of dozens of important enzymes, is a component of the insulin that regulates our energy supply, and works with red blood cells to transport waste carbon dioxide from body tissue to the lungs, where it is expelled. Zinc is also vital to the production of the RNA and DNA that oversee the division, growth, and repair of the body's cells; helps preserve our sense of taste and smell; and aids in wound healing.

The RDA for zinc is 15 milligrams, not to exceed 40 milligrams per day for adults over eighteen years of age. Women who are pregnant may want to take an additional 5 milligrams of zinc daily, and women who are breastfeeding an extra 10 milligrams daily.

Choose Foods That Provide Zinc

Dietary sources of zinc include beef, herring, seafood, pork, poultry, milk, soybeans, and whole grains.

"Nothing lifts me out of a bad mood better than a hard workout on my treadmill. It never fails. Exercise is nothing short of a miracle."

—Cher

Start Your Day on a Treadmill

A treadmill is a good option for indoor running (or walking) and can be done at home, at a gym, or club. There are new indoor treadmills coming to market all the time. The best indoor treadmill is the one that works for you. Experiment with several before you hone in on one, and be receptive to trying new ones that show up in your gym.

Running on treadmills is recommended when you have no choice and you don't want to miss a workout. The treadmill's convenience is wonderful, but ultimately it will not help you train for long-distance running. Those in training for a marathon still need to do a large percentage of running on roads, particularly with those all-important long runs. As you run indoors, remember to focus on your form. When you exercise, proper posture and technique are essential to maximizing your effort and avoiding injury. Many runners respect the importance of posture and mechanics when doing outside sports but give little thought to these when exercising indoors on equipment.

HOW TO COMPUTE YOUR MILES PER HOUR

Pace is the number of minutes it takes to travel 1 mile. To determine your pace, divide 60 by your speed in miles per hour. For example: If your treadmill speed equals 3.5 mph, divide 60 by 3.5. You are running a 17-minute mile.

"Basketball is an endurance sport, and you have to learn to control your breath; that's the essence of yoga, too. So, I consciously began using yoga techniques in my practice and playing. I think yoga helped reduce the number and severity of injuries I suffered. As preventative medicine, it's unequaled."

—Kareem Abdul-Jabbar

Strengthen Your Wrists with a One-Arm Side Balance

To do a one-arm side balance (Vasisthasana) come into downward-facing dog. Place your right hand at the midline of your body (halfway to your left hand and in line with it) and the outside of your right foot on the floor. Lift your left hand off the floor and place it on your left hip, as you place your left foot over the right foot and turn the body to face sideways. Stack your ankles, hips, and shoulders. Stretch actively through your feet and lengthen the front of your body from the pubis to the sternum. Keep your head in line with your spine. Extend your left arm up perpendicular to the floor and press down through your right hand, lengthening up through your right arm. Lift your right hip up, so it does not sag down. Stay for several breaths and then come back into downward-facing dog, bend your knees, and come down. Rest, and then repeat on the other side.

You can also try placing your feet against the wall for additional support and help with alignment. Or, instead of bringing your upper leg on top of the lower leg, place your upper leg in front of your lower leg. Bend your leg and turn your foot to face your lower foot. Press through both feet.

The benefits of the one-arm side pose include the following:

- It develops coordination.
- It strengthens the wrists.
- It tones the lower spine.

"What started as a promise to my sister turned into a global movement."

—Nancy G. Brinker, founder of the Susan G. Komen Race for the Cure®

Walk for a Cause

You can get in shape for a good cause and earn money for medical research teams and exercise at the same time. Join forces with the Leukemia Foundation for a Cure or the Fight Against Breast Cancer or the American Heart Association and walk to raise money for medical research. Here are several walks that may have local opportunities, and if not, you can create the first walk in your area!

- **Walk for breast cancer.** Roughly, 182,000 women receive a breast cancer diagnosis each year. A staggering 43,300 will die. Not only women, but also men, get breast cancer. Find a variety of ways to help fight this dreaded disease and multiple websites with information by logging onto *www.breastcancersite.org*.
- **Participate in a Relay for Life.** Held by the American Cancer Society these overnight events are held in cities and towns across the country. Check out the Relay for Life website at *www.relayforlife .org* and learn how you can form a team and participate in a relay in your area.
- **Join the Asthma Walk to help find a cure.** More than 20 million Americans have asthma and nearly 4,000 die every year. Pollutants in the environment pose increased health hazards to asthma sufferers. Go to *www.lungusa.org* for more information.

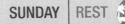

"If you're going through hell, keep going."

—Winston Churchill

Take a Hike

Stress evokes the "fight or flight" reaction by releasing stress hormones into the body designed to give us sudden, quick reactions, extra strength, and endurance. When we don't respond to the stress response by moving quickly, using our strength, or taking advantage of the added endurance, our bodies are all geared up with no outlet for that energy. Muscles stay tense. Blood pressure stays high. Breathing stays shallow. Cortisol and adrenaline course through the body, causing all kinds of problems when the body doesn't react the way it is being programmed to react.

Because your body is primed to physically react when feeling stressed, taking a brisk walk around the block (or two, or three) can provide instant relief, particularly if you hustle. Once your brain gets the message that you are, in fact, moving quickly, it responds by returning to equilibrium and releasing beta endorphins that will further calm your body.

In other words, exercise makes the obsolete "fight or flight" stress response relevant again. It lets your body respond the way it is trying to respond. Rather than sitting and fuming (what caveperson ever did that in response to a charging predator?), you are getting up and moving. "Ahh . . ." the body responds. "this is what I want to do!"

And you are *finally* able to relax.

"Yet this is health: To have a body functioning so perfectly that when its few simple needs are met it never calls attention to its own existence."

—Bertha Stuart Dyment

Use Micro-Plants in Vegetable Smoothies

Micro-plants consisting of blue-green algae, chlorella, spirulina, wheat grass, and barley grass contain more vitamins and minerals than kale and broccoli. They are an excellent source of two important phytochemicals: chlorophyll and lycopene. Micro-plants, commercially known as green foods, contain a concentrated combination of phytochemicals, vitamins, minerals, bioflavonoids, proteins, amino acids, essential fatty acids, enzymes, coenzymes, and fiber. They support your body's ability to detoxify heavy metals, pesticides, and other toxins, plus boost your immunity to disease. Here's a very green smoothie that combines a variety of greens for the very best benefits! Spinach, kale, and wheatgrass are packed with vitamins and minerals that work hard to maintain your health.

VERY GREEN SMOOTHIE

Recipe Yields: 3–4 cups
1 cup spinach
2 kale leaves
1 cup wheatgrass
1 celery stalk
½ lemon, peeled
1 garlic clove
2 cups chamomile tea

1. Combine spinach, kale, wheatgrass, celery, lemon, garlic, and 1 cup of tea in a blender and blend until thoroughly combined.
2. Add remaining 1 cup of tea as needed while blending until desired consistency is achieved.

PER 1 CUP SERVING: Calories 16 | Fat 0g | Protein 1g | Sodium 25mg | Fiber 1g | Carbohydrates 3g

"When your muscles are challenged to lift something heavier than they are used to, they respond by growing stronger to meet the challenge."

—Shirley S. Archer, fitness professional, Stanford University School of Medicine

Add Plyometric Jumping Lunges

Like jumping squats and lateral pushes, jumping lunges are plyometric exercises that involve using your own body weight to build strength. You will want to be very comfortable doing lunges before you attempt these, and, as always, you should start slowly and build up strength before adding them to your daily workout. Here's how to do jumping lunges:

1. Start with you feet hip width part, as you would for a regular lunge. Bend your knees slightly and do a small jump, landing at the bottom of a lunge, with one leg bent at the knee and the other stretched out behind you.
2. From the bottom of a lunge, jump up evenly with both legs, switch your lead leg while in the air, and land in a lunge with your other leg forward.
3. Upon landing, stabilize the lower body then repeat this lunge on the other side. Try to make this exercise fluid when jumping from one lunge to the next.

You may find it helpful to swing your arms from one lunge to the next. This can also be done without any arm swing to further challenge your leg power. Try making each repetition fluid and controlled, with soft landings from one jump to the next.

*"Everybody seized upon a bit of the beast.
The Sultan claimed the liver, which, when dried and powdered,
is worth twice its weight in gold as medicine."*

—Isabella Bird

Eat Copper-Rich Foods

Copper is found in all tissues in the body but is concentrated in the brain, heart, kidney, and liver. It helps the body make hemoglobin (needed to carry oxygen to red blood cells) and red blood cells by aiding in the absorption of iron. Copper is part of many enzymes in the body and helps produce energy in cells. In addition, copper helps make hormones that regulate a variety of body functions, including heartbeat, blood pressure, and wound healing. Most deficiencies are due to a genetic problem or from too much zinc.

Copper is found mostly in organ meats, especially liver, and in seafood, nuts, and seeds. It can also be found in poultry, legumes, and dark green leafy vegetables. Here's a recipe for pesto that contains copper-rich nuts, as well as other nutrients:

BASIL PINE NUT PESTO

Serve over greens, pasta, or vegetables. Substitute pumpkin seeds, walnuts, or hazelnuts for pine nuts. Cilantro, parsley, or arugula can be used in place of basil. For variation, add sun-dried tomatoes, black olives, capers, lemon rind, coriander, mushrooms, or artichoke for a different flavor.

Serves 6
¼ **cup pine nuts**
¼ **cup walnuts**
2 **cloves garlic**
1 **teaspoon lemon juice**
1½ **tablespoons sweet white miso**
¼ **cup extra virgin olive oil**
¼ **cup spring water**
2 **teaspoons tahini**
2 **cups basil leaves, loosely packed**

BASIL PINE NUT PESTO *Continued*

1. Roast pine nuts and walnuts separately in a dry skillet until lightly browned, about 8 minutes each. Grind pine nuts and walnuts in a blender or food processor and pour into a small bowl.
2. Combine garlic, lemon juice, miso, olive oil, water, and tahini in blender and process. Chop basil leaves finely, add to blender, and process. Add nuts and blend until combined. Slowly blend more water or oil into sauce until desired consistency is reached. Store, covered, in the refrigerator for up to 3 days.

PER SERVING: Calories 170 | **Fat** 17g | **Sodium** 85mg | **Carbohydrate** 4g | **Fiber** 1g | **Protein** 2g

"Another hour on the erg; after a while, this monastic existence becomes familiar and almost comforting. I feel like every day is spent more carefully; when I do go out with friends, the experiences are much more meaningful, thanks to the structure placed upon my life."

—Alessandra Phillips

Add an Ergometer Workout

One popular cross-training machine is the ergometer, or rowing machine. As scullers have known for centuries, rowing is a terrific all-body exercise, strengthening your back, buttocks, and legs and developing your shoulders and arms. Rowing involves a two-stroke movement referred to as the drive and the recovery, which together produce a smooth and continuous action. It's important to follow good form on a rowing machine, so make sure you ask your health club to show you how to use it properly. This is another highly beneficial activity to do on a rest day. It strengthens the hips, buttocks, and upper body while sparing your legs.

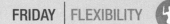
"When you inhale, you are taking the strength from God. When you exhale, it represents the service you are giving to the world."

—B.K.S. Iyengar

Improve the Range and Flexibility of Your Hips with the Lunge Pose

The lunge pose begins on all fours. Look forward, and bring your right leg forward, planting your right foot between your hands. Place your fingertips alongside your right foot. Spread the toes and balls of your feet, and lift the arches. Your right shin is perpendicular to the floor, with the knee over the heel. Extend your left leg from the hip to the heel with the toes tucked under. Lift the back thigh away from the floor slightly, to ensure that the thighbone is feeding into the socket, rather than hanging out of the socket (hanging from the hip joint is detrimental to the health of the joint and its surrounding ligaments and tendons). Ground your right foot and toes of your left foot. Maintain the extension of the spine from the tailbone to the crown of your head. Press into your fingertips and stretch your arms up into the shoulder sockets to support your upper body. Be in the pose for several breaths. Then release and repeat on the left side.

You can also try bending the back knee and resting it on the floor. This action will increase the opening and lengthening of the groin and the front of the back thigh. Place blocks at an appropriate height under the hands to increase comfort and ease in the pose and to maintain the length of the arms and the extension of the spine out of the pelvis.

The benefits of the lunge pose include the following:

- It improves range of motion and flexibility of the hips.
- It stretches and opens the groin and the psoas muscle.
- It warms up and prepares the body for backbends by opening the groin.

"There are really only two plays: Romeo and Juliet,
and put the darn ball in the basket."

—Abe Lemons

Play a Pickup Game of Basketball

Playing pick-up basketball provides a way to have fun while getting aerobic exercise. It's a great cardiovascular workout; all that running and jumping really works your heart and lungs. One moment, you're on one side of the court passing the ball, moving left and right and forward and back trying to get the ball through the hoop. The next moment, you are sprinting down to the other end of the court as possession of the ball changes hands. Though this may seem like continuous movement, your heart rate fluctuates a great deal depending on what is occurring at any given moment in the game—and you are strengthening your muscles, increasing your flexibility, and burning fat. Additionally, you are increasing your speed and agility, building endurance. It's also a way to hang out with friends, or make new ones. All in all, pick-up basketball on an otherwise lazy Saturday afternoon provides so many health and relaxation benefits that we can't think of single reason not to pick up the phone and rally your buddies.

Calories Burned: 460 per hour.

IT'S ALSO REALLY, REALLY GOOD FOR YOUR KIDS

If you've got children who can join in the game, playing pick-up basketball offers opportunities to teach them teamwork, sportsmanship, and unbridled enthusiasm. Have a blast and use the game as a teachable moment by modeling and reinforcing the desired behaviors. You can even opt to let your kid be the captain.

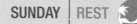

"The healthy, the strong individual, is the one who asks for help when he needs it. Whether he has an abscess on his knee or in his soul."

—Rona Barrett

Create a Personal Stress Management Portfolio

Because the word stress can mean so many things to so many different people, it's logical that before any one individual—that means you—can put an effective stress management plan into practice, a Personal Stress Profile is essential. By determining the unique stressors you experience in your life, your personality's stress-related tendencies, and how you personally tend to cope with stress, you can design a Stress Management Portfolio that really works for you.

For example, someone who is physically drained by too much interaction with people may not be helped by strategies that encourage increased social activities with friends. Someone else who is stressed by the lack of a support system might find profound benefit in increased social activity. Some people are deeply calmed by meditation; others find it excruciating. Some people find assertiveness training a relief, but a naturally assertive type might benefit more from learning to sit back and let other people handle things.

You can think of your Personal Stress Profile, or PSP, as something like a business proposal. You are the business, and the business isn't operating at peak efficiency. Your PSP is a picture of the business as a whole and the specific nature of all the factors that are keeping the business from performing as well as it could. With PSP in hand, you can effectively create your own Stress Management Portfolio. Before you know it, you'll be running smoothly, efficiently, and productively (not to mention happily).

Once you've identified the problems causing your stress and have a game plan in the form of your Stress Management Portfolio, create an action list of things that you can do to begin to resolve your stress on a daily basis.

*"The breakfast slimes, angel food cake, doughnuts and coffee,
white bread and gravy cannot build an enduring nation."*

—Martin H. Fischer

Start Your Day with a Delicious Smoothie

On days you're in a rush, blending a nutritious smoothie is a great way to provide yourself, and your family, with a potent mix of protein and vitamins that will get everyone off to a good start. Here's a recipe that's nutritious, delicious, and will please everyone:

STRAWBERRY BREAKFAST SMOOTHIE

Recipe Yields: 3–4 cups

1 cup romaine lettuce
2 pints strawberries
2 bananas, peeled
1 cup strawberry kefir
1 cup ice

1. Combine romaine, strawberries, bananas, and kefir in a blender and blend until thoroughly combined.
2. Add ice as needed while blending until desired consistency is achieved.

PER 1 CUP SERVING: Calories 136 | **Fat** 1g | **Protein** 5g | **Sodium** 35mg | **Fiber** 5g | **Carbohydrates** 30g

"Suffer the pain of discipline or suffer the pain of regret."

—Unknown

Add a Platform Jump to Your Workout

Having something in front of you to jump up onto, such as a platform, adds a couple of elements to your workout. It adds a competitive element either with yourself or with a training partner in that it challenges you to jump higher to get up onto the platform. It also adds a measurable element that makes jumping much more interesting. Maybe your fist platform jump is only eight inches high, but two weeks later you are now jumping onto a platform that is twelve inches high.

1. Stand in front of a platform, bench, or step (between roughly eight and twenty inches high depending on the desired level of difficulty) that has a stable surface.
2. Swing your arms down and back while bending at the knees and hips, again similar to a squat.
3. Swing your arms up and burst off the ground, jumping up onto the platform and landing with a light and controlled manner. You may choose to step down in the beginning and repeat the exercise again, or you can jump back to where you started with a smooth and controlled landing.

The progression is to increase the height of the platform as you develop more power. Remember how important the arm swing is for height. If you find you are having trouble jumping up onto a certain height, try using a bigger and faster arm swing. The arm swing tends to be forgotten about when you're focused on jumping onto something that is raised up.

Once you are comfortable with jumping onto the platform, it is time to jump back down. You can do this in two ways. First, jump down while facing forward, again landing in a squat. Once you are comfortable with the height, jump off the platform moving backward, landing in the same spot you took off from.

"We choose and sculpt how our ever-changing minds will work, we choose who we will be the next moment in a very real sense, and these choices are left embossed in physical form on our material selves."

—Dr. Mike Merzenich

Become an Optimist!

Neuroscientists have discovered that people who have a more cheerful disposition and are more prone to optimism generally show more brain activity in their left prefrontal cortex. This is the part of your brain that has the most control over brain function and that processes feelings. The more activity in that region, the happier you tend to be. In fact, behavioral scientists have observed very interesting differences between optimists and pessimists. In general, they have found that optimists:

- Attribute good events to themselves in terms of permanence, citing their traits and abilities as the cause, and bad events as transient (using terms such as "sometimes" or "lately" to describe them.)
- See setbacks as surmountable and particular to a single external problem, resulting from temporary problems or other people, not themselves.
- Lead happy, rich, fulfilled lives.
- Spend the least amount of time alone, and the most time socializing.
- Maintain healthier relationships.
- Have better health habits.
- Have stronger immune systems.
- Live longer than pessimists.

Optimism involves highly desirable cognitive, emotional, and motivational components. Optimists tend to have better moods, to be more persevering and successful, and to experience better physical health. So, come on, look on the bright side of life and be happier!

"Cross country skiing is great if you live in a small country."

—Steven Wright

Add NordicTrack Workouts to Your Endurance Training

If there's no snow for cross-country skiing, another machine that provides a great upper- and lower-body workout is the NordicTrack. The NordicTrack and other machines that simulate cross-country skiing can be very effective in improving your coordination and balance while they work to increase your stamina, build muscles, and improve your overall aerobic fitness. Keep in mind that time spent on the NordicTrack is time spent readying yourself to actually go cross-country skiing the next time the weather permits.

"Sun salutations can energize and warm you,
even on the darkest, coldest winter day."

—Carol Krucoff

Sample a Yogi's Favorite Smoothie

Hot, or not, yoga can be a powerful workout. Replenish your body and refresh your senses with this sweet blend of melons, citrus, and berries. A definite "Yum!" to follow your "Om!"

FROM OM TO YUM

Recipe Yields: 3–4 cups
1 cup watercress
½ honeydew, rind and seeds removed
2 tangerines, peeled
1 cucumber, peeled
1 cup Greek-style yogurt

1. Combine watercress, honeydew, tangerines, cucumber, and ½ cup yogurt in a blender and blend until thoroughly combined.
2. Add remaining ½ cup yogurt as needed while blending until desired consistency is achieved.

PER 1 CUP SERVING: Calories 120 | **Fat** 0g | **Protein** 7g | **Sodium** 58mg | **Fiber** 2g | **Carbohydrates** 24g

"Frustration is the first step towards improvement. I have no incentive to improve if I'm content with what I can do and if I'm completely satisfied with my pace, distance, and form as a runner. It's only when I face frustration and use it to fuel my dedication that I feel myself moving forwards."

—John Bingham

Play Racquetball

One of the great things about this sport is that you'll burn a lot of calories even when you're starting out. A 150-pound person can expect to burn 500 calories at the beginning and push this into the 800s as he becomes more agile and gains stamina. In this interval-style sport that provides aerobic and anaerobic benefits, you'll run nearly 2 miles an hour and you won't even notice it—although your heart, waistline, and metabolism will!

HEART WORKOUT

Racquetball is also a great workout for your heart. Players typically work at 75 percent to 85 percent of their maximum heart rate consistently. During the course of a 20-minute game, each player will run an average of about two miles. *Men's Health* says that players burn about 794 calories per hour.

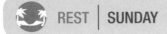

"Your innermost sense of self, of who you are, is inseparable from stillness. This is the I Am that is deeper than name and form."

—Eckhart Tolle

Find Your Own Om

The traditional mantra of yoga meditation is the sound/word "Om." The sound is meant to imitate the sound of the universe, from which everything originated and of which everything is a part. Some people think of it as the sound of God. By saying/making this sound, many practitioners believe you can feel a connection with the universe, and that is the philosophical basis of yoga (and Hinduism)—we are all one with the universe; all matter, all energy, everything is connected; everything ultimately merges together; beneath the surface of reality, which we experience with our senses, all is really just one. Some people who practice meditation like to use the mantra "One" instead of the mantra "Om" because it more directly evokes, to them, this idea.

If you choose to use "Om" as your meditation mantra, when you are relaxed and ready to begin your slow, rhythmical breathing, say "Om" slowly, as you exhale. Begin in the back of your throat, with your mouth slightly open. Allow the sound to vibrate in your mouth and become an "M" sound as you slowly close your mouth. Practice often, and the "Om" will soon resonate through your body.

If you prefer another sound, that's fine. Simply repeat your chosen sound with each exhalation for five minutes on your first time out, then increase the time in meditation as instructed. Meditation should be an energizing spiritual reinforcement, which is important for getting stress under control. If you are feeding your spiritual side, you tend to be less stressed out by the less important things in life.

"Nearly one-third of the U.S. population is walking around in a state of chronic mild dehydration. . . . If a person is dehydrated up to two percent, a proper fluid balance can be restored by taking in fluids within six hours. Once a person is past three percent it can take up to twenty-four hours to restore balance."

—Susan Kleiner, PhD, RD, specialist in high performance nutrition

Make Hydration a Priority

Water is essential to cellular function. Water regulates body temperature, lubricates joints, assists in elimination of wastes, and protects body tissues. Approximately 60 percent of an adult's body weight is water. Of all the nutrients, water is most essential to survival. Every system in your body depends on water to function. It makes sense that systems are affected by dehydration. Your muscles can't perform effectively if you're dehydrated. Thirst is not a good indicator of hydration. We often become thirsty far beyond the point when we should have started to replenish fluids. And, as we age our thirst mechanism loses sensitivity.

Here's a "fluid plan" to make sure you get your daily eight to ten cups of water:

- Measure out eight to ten cups so you can visualize the amount.
- Carry a water bottle with you all day. Know how much it holds so you know your consumption when you empty it.
- Drink bottled water in the car.
- Drink in the morning, at your desk, lunch, mid-afternoon, and at dinner.
- Carry your water bottle with you at the gym or whenever you exercise.
- For every fifteen minutes of exercise, drink one additional cup.
- If you're a skier, walker, or long distance runner, carry a back pouch with water. Regularly wash and disinfect your water bottles and pouches.

"My dream is to become a farmer. Just a Bohemian guy pulling up his own sweet potatoes for dinner."

—Lenny Kravitz

Rev Up with a Sweet Potato Smoothie

Even though being an avid athlete means focusing on the healthiest foods that provide ideal nutrition calorie for calorie, cravings for sweet treats creep up every once in a while. Calm those cravings with combinations like this that satisfy with sound nutrition!

SWEET POTATO SMOOTHIE

Recipe Yields: 3–4 cups
½ cup walnuts
2 cups purified water
1 cup spinach
1 sweet potato, peeled and cut for blender's ability (if you don't have a blender capable of handling a raw sweet potato, cook it for 2-3 minutes in your microwave first).
1 teaspoon pumpkin pie spice

1. Combine walnuts and 1 cup of water in a blender and blend until emulsified and no walnut bits remain.
2. Add spinach, sweet potato, pumpkin pie spice, and remaining 1 cup of water while blending until desired consistency is achieved.

PER 1 CUP SERVING: Calories 127 | **Fat** 10g | **Protein** 3g | **Sodium** 19mg | **Fiber** 2g | **Carbohydrates** 9g

---

WALNUTS FOR ATHLETIC PERFORMANCE

Just ¼ cup of walnuts contains almost 100 percent of your daily value of omega-3s. Not only a tasty, protein-packed morsel, the walnut helps athletes perform at their best by improving circulation and heart health, controlling blood pressure, providing essential amino acids, and acting as a powerful antioxidant.

"Spanish cooking is drier, more singular, not as diffused. It's about one ingredient tasting very good, like tossing sardines with garlic and parsley and leaving it alone. Even when chefs riff on it, they don't put a lot on the plate."

—Anya Von Bremzen

Add Coenzyme Q10

Anything that benefits heart health, particularly cholesterol levels, blood flow, and blood pressure, is also vital for your brain. CoQ10 has been shown to be useful in alleviating the effects of abnormalities involving the heart's ability to contract and pump blood effectively, such as congestive heart failure and a number of heart muscle diseases. Coenzyme Q10 also appears to protect vitamin E, which helps prevent the oxidation of low-density lipoprotein (LDL, or "bad" cholesterol). It's believed that oxidized LDL can lead to plaque buildup, clogged arteries, and an increased risk of heart attack or stroke. CoQ10 may reduce the ability of blood to clot, thereby decreasing the chance of a blood clot getting stuck in a clogged artery and causing a heart attack or stroke. Other heart-related conditions for which CoQ10 supplementation shows promise include hypertension and heart valve replacement.

Supplements are readily available, but consult with your doctor before adding them to your daily supplements.

> **CHOOSE FOODS WITH COENZYME Q10**
>
> To bulk up on CoQ10 eat sardines, mackerel, nuts, organ meats, beef, broccoli, chicken, oranges, salmon, or trout.

"I ran on the treadmill some and ran on the elliptical. I've done the stair-master the past couple of days, ridden the bike and shot around."

—Jodi Howell

Use the Elliptical Trainer to Strengthen Leg Muscles

For those of you who hate the treadmill, but want a full-body workout on an aerobic machine, check out the elliptical trainer. By combining cross-country skiing with climbing stairs and walking, the machine is able to provide an excellent cardiovascular workout without hurting your joints. The motion works all of the major muscle groups in your legs and offers the option to move backward and really focus on those glutes. Another great benefit of the machine is that you can adjust the program to your strength level, which allows both beginners and more advanced athletes to get a solid workout as they increase the resistance.

OR YOU COULD JUST GO THE STAIR CLIMBING ROUTE

You can also add to your leg strength and endurance with stair climbing. Find a building tall enough to allow you to climb for two minutes at a moderate pace (between simple climbing and a sprint). If two minutes on the stairs is too much at first, start with one minute and build up. Once you can do two minutes, repeat six to eight times once a week. If you don't have access to a tall building, perhaps there is a stadium you can use for stair running. Go up and down five or six times once a week.

"If you understand the force of intelligence in the body, its mechanical operation and structure, you can work on any part of the body you can reach with your hands."

—Lauren Berry

Learn to Self-Massage

If you learn about acupressure, Swedish massage, reflexology, and many other techniques, you can perform massage on yourself. You can massage your own neck, scalp, face, hands, feet, legs, arms, and torso. Many yoga postures also result in internal and external massage by bending the body in certain ways against itself or by using the pressure of the floor against certain parts of the body.

Treat yourself to a variety of massages until you find the particular methods that deliver the best results in decreasing muscular or joint pain and in providing relaxation. Then, create your own unique brand of massage and use it on all the areas of your body that you can reach—head, neck, shoulders, arms, hands, chest, stomach, lower back, legs, and feet.

Experiment with oils to see which ones feel or smell particularly good to you. Some oils are invigorating, like peppermint, while others can be restive, like lavender. You can also use pain-relieving creams if your muscles feel particularly stressed.

Follow your self-massage with a warm bath filled with Epsom salts, and you'll likely wake up the next day feeling refreshed and invigorated.

"I was always singing and dancing for my mother when I wasn't glued to the television watching I Love Lucy *or* The Carol Burnett Show. *"*

—Debra Messing

Dance the Night Away

Even if you have two left feet, turn on your CD player or put your iPod in its docking station and start moving. Whether it's in your bedroom or your living room or a local club or studio, dancing is great for your over-all health because you move quickly and use all of your limbs. The funny thing about dancing, too, is that all you really need is a sense of rhythm and an enjoyment of music—you can be good at it no matter what your size or shape. Dancing also happens to be an incredible cardio work-out and can help you release stress and tone your whole body through movement. Even if you start out with two left feet, after a handful of weekends out dancing at a club or in a scheduled course, you'll start to have some rhythm and more confidence out on the dance floor. Dancing is a win-win activity: It's exercise—and it's fun!

BURN, BABY, BURN

Go out for an evening of dance and try to put in at least an hour on the floor. Because whether you have enough stamina to keep it up for an hour or you need to slow down your moves from time to time, you'll be lighting those metabolic fires. Take a look at what a 150-pound person burns on average for an hour for these different dancing styles:

- **Aerobic dance/nightclubbing:** 442 calories
- **Fast Ballroom:** 374 calories
- **Ballet, Jazz, or Tap:** 326 calories
- **Medium-Speed Ballroom (Polka, Line):** 306 calories
- **Slow-Speed Ballroom (Waltz, Tango, Mambo):** 204 calories

*"The yoga mat is a good place to turn when talk therapy
and antidepressants aren't enough."*

—Amy Weintraub

Weather Hard Times by Practicing Yoga

Yoga is also a powerful, holistic, transformational tool that calms and focuses the mind and develops innate intelligence and awareness. The postures, breath awareness, and relaxation techniques develop your natural intuitive intelligence, and help your mind to focus on one thing at a time instead of jumping around like a hyper monkey. When the mind is focused, the nervous, circulatory, and respiratory systems respond by slowing down. The body and mind start to relax. You feel calmer, think more clearly, and feel centered and grounded. Over time, the mind and the intelligence are able to spread throughout the body, focusing on many points at one time. This is *meditation.*

As the mind quiets, the body opens to release unnecessary tension and long-held emotions. The emotions become balanced and moderate. The body develops balanced strength, and with strength comes flexibility and a stable core. You experience emotional equanimity and poise, like a tree that sways in the breeze but always come back to center. Life will always have its sunny days and stormy, windy times, but yoga creates a strong foundation with which you can endure life's unpredictable weather.

"I did not become a vegetarian for my health,
I did it for the health of the chickens."

—Isaac Bashevis Singer

Grow Your Own Organic Produce and Herbs

If you have access to a deck, a roof, or even a small patch of ground, you can grow your own produce. Herbs can be grown on a windowsill, and tomato and bell pepper plants can thrive in a container on a balcony or patio. Hanging containers are a great way to grow smaller vegetable and fruit plants or herbs without taking up any floor space.

The best thing about backyard organic gardens is that you're in control of the fertilizers, pesticides, herbicides, and growing aids you use. You can opt for all-natural alternatives that will not harm the soil, animals, or your family. Limit weeds and reduce the need for chemical-laden weed killers by weeding regularly and using natural or reclaimed ground cover between your food plants. Store-bought weed prevention products are also available in ready-to-use natural and organic versions, including Preen Organic Vegetable Garden Weed, Perfectly Natural Weed N Grass Killer, Weed Pharm Organic Weed Control, and Green Light Organic Spot Weeder. Here's a list of resources that can help you get started.

ORGANIC GARDENING RESOURCES

For complete details and lots of encouragement on growing your own backyard or patio organic garden, check out these helpful websites:

- *www.the-organic-gardener.com*
- *www.your-vegetable-gardening-helper.com*
- *www.organicgardening.com*, the companion site to the magazine *Organic Gardening*

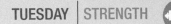

"We either make ourselves miserable or we make ourselves strong.
The amount of work is the same."

—Carlos Castaneda

Add a Kettle Bell Swing (or Double-Arm Swing)

A kettle bell is a weighted ball with a handle that can be held in the hand and lifted, swung, flipped, and thrown. You can move it in an infinite amount of angles and directions, which makes it an interesting and dynamic tool to train with.

The foundational movement of kettle bell training is what's called a kettle bell swing. It is very much like a vertical jump and an upper-body plyometric combined into one exercise.

1. Begin with your feet hip width apart or slightly wider while holding the kettle bell or weight in front of you with two hands.
2. As you move your hips back down into your squat, the weight will swing back slightly between your legs.
3. As the weight you are using begins to swing forward and up, you must drive your heels and legs down into the floor and burst upward.
4. The weight should propel upward rather than being lifted solely by your shoulder muscles. Think of your hips like an engine and your arms like ropes with hooks on the ends.
5. Power is generated from the ground up through the legs, forcing the bell up and away from you. The bell has to be slowed down with control on the way down and redirected to travel back up again. The same exercise can be performed with one hand at a time as well.

"Oh, sweet sorrow, the time you borrow,
will you be here when i wake up tomorrow?"

—Katherine Wolf

Ask Your Doctor about SAMe

SAMe (pronounced "Sammy") is a form of the amino acid methionine that occurs naturally in the body and is used for many essential functions, including making cartilage. SAMe appears to increase the levels of certain neurotransmitters, and may thereby affect moods and emotions. In nine studies, SAMe compared favorably with antidepressant drugs, including imipramine, amitryptaline, and clomipramine. Some researchers have found that SAMe supplementation has improved mood disorders, without the side effects of other antidepressants (such as weight gain, headaches, sleep disturbances, and sexual dysfunction). And, SAMe works faster than some prescription antidepressants, often in four to ten days compared with two to six weeks for drugs.

Don't Take SAMe If . . .

When it comes to taking SAMe as a relief from psychological problems, never attempt to self-medicate—always consult your doctor. Absolutely do not take SAMe when you are already taking drugs for bipolar depression, obsessive compulsive disorder, or addictive tendencies, as it has been known to worsen symptoms.

"People who had high daily levels of sitting (7.4 hours or more) were significantly more likely to be overweight or obese than those who reported low daily sitting levels (less than 4.7 hours a day)."

—*International Journal of Obesity and Related Metabolic Disorders*

Add Variety to Stair Workouts

Walking or running up stairs is an inexpensive and effective way to work on strength and endurance. Here are a few ideas that you can use to changeup your workouts, bolstering your overall endurance:

- Add stair lunges: To do stair lunges simply walk up stairs taking two- or three-step lunges at a time. Doing so puts your legs at a mechanical disadvantage, which forces them to become stronger to overcome this disadvantage.
- Increase the number of step strides: If you have mastered taking two-step lunges at a time, move it to three steps. That one extra step makes a big difference and will challenge almost anyone, with perhaps the exception of very tall people. Don't go as high as four-step lunges as they move you into the danger zone.
- Put your hands behind your head: This challenges your balance and increases the work your legs have to do.
- Go up sideways: Stand parallel to the stairs and lift your left or right leg, whichever you've chosen to work first, to mount the stairs. Do sets with both sides and this will help you identify which leg is weaker so you can focus on improving strength on that side. Start with one-step lifts until you feel ready to add that second step.
- Do crossover stair lunges: Once you've mastered the two- to three-step lunges, add crossover lunges. It's as simple as crossing your legs as you go up, moving from side-to-side, and with rotation. These will improve your dynamic flexibility and strength balance. Start with one-step lunges until you're confident with this move.

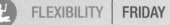

"When asked what gift he wanted for his birthday,
the yogi replied: 'I wish no gifts, only presence.'"

—Author Unknown

Increase Your Stamina with Ashtanga (Power) Yoga

Most yoga taught in the United States is a form of Hatha Yoga, which is comprised of physical postures, breathing techniques, relaxation, and meditation. Hatha Yoga is the umbrella under which most of the sub-specialties of yoga fall. What makes the styles different from each other is their emphasis and technique.

Ashtanga Yoga is a dynamic, fast-paced, challenging series of sequential poses linked together by *ujjayi* breath (a specific breathing technique that sounds like Darth Vader) and a flow of postures called *vinyasa*. It is a heat-producing, detoxifying, and flowing practice that creates strength and flexibility and increases stamina. It is a style that appeals to athletically inclined individuals who enjoy intense and challenging exercise. The system is based on six series, each increasing in difficulty.

An Americanized hybrid of Ashtanga Yoga is *Power Yoga,* a term originating from Beryl Bender Birch, Ashtanga Yoga teacher and author of *Power Yoga.* Most Power Yoga is a vigorous, flowing series of postures based upon the Ashtanga Yoga system. Many health clubs have embraced Power Yoga as a transition from aerobics to yoga.

IF FIREFIGHTERS DO IT . . .

Firefighters in Los Altos, California, originally incorporated yoga into their fitness routine to increase their strength and flexibility. But after eighteen months, they've discovered additional benefits. The team has become closer and they have more fun together. They've also noticed that they are calmer and more connected during emergencies.

"All men are created equal, then a few become firemen."

—Anonymous

Become an Asset to Your Community

One fabulous way to become an asset to your community, provided you can qualify, is to help support the first line of defense that protects your community in the case of a fire. Pledge your time, hard work, and willpower to your local volunteer firefighting force. Check out *www.nvfc.org* for more information on the volunteer force.

If that's a tad too strenuous or too time-consuming, volunteer to participate as a part of your town's disaster relief team. When a natural disaster has hit or is about to hit your hometown, you can help out. Whether it's building sandbag walls or volunteering at evacuation centers, you can play an important role in everyone else's safety.

Or, get involved in your community's Citizens Corps Council. The council keeps communities safe from disasters, terrorism, and crime. A component of the U.S. Freedom Corps and coordinated by the Department of Homeland Security, the council encourages local citizens to participate in setting up programs, developing plans of action, locating local resources, and assessing threats to their communities. For more information, visit *www.citizencorps.gov*.

The point is to spend your time productively, get some physical exercise, make some new friends, and be an asset to your community.

DISASTER PREPARATION

Prepare for a disaster. Check out the Department of Homeland Security's disaster preparedness website and find ideas to prepare your kids and your business for unexpected disaster. See *www.ready.gov*.

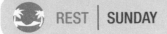

"Sleeping alone, except under doctor's orders, does much harm. Children will tell you how lonely it is sleeping alone. If possible, you should always sleep with someone you love. You both recharge your mutual batteries free of charge."

—Marlene Dietrich

Make It Easier to Sleep

If you are having trouble sleeping, try these suggestions:

- Don't drink or eat anything with caffeine after lunch. That includes coffee, tea, cola, and many other sodas (check the label); certain over-the-counter pain medications and cold medications (check the label); stimulants designed to keep you awake; and even cocoa and chocolate.
- Eat a healthy, light, low-fat, low-carbohydrate dinner. Fresh fruits and vegetables, whole grains instead of refined grains, and low-fat protein like fish, chicken, beans, and tofu will help your body to be in a calmer, more balanced state come bedtime. Avoid high-fat, overly processed foods in the evening.
- For an evening snack, eat foods high in tryptophan, an amino acid that encourages the body to produce serotonin, a chemical that helps you to sleep. Foods high in tryptophan include milk, turkey, peanut butter, rice, tuna, dates, figs, and yogurt. A light snack about thirty to sixty minutes before bedtime that includes any of these foods can help promote restful sleep.
- Don't drink alcohol in the evening. While many people have a drink thinking it will help them get to sleep, alcohol actually disrupts sleep patterns, making your sleep less restful. Alcohol may also increase snoring and sleep apnea.
- Get enough exercise during the day. A well-exercised body will fall asleep faster, sleep longer, and sleep more productively.

"Up to the age of forty eating is beneficial. After forty, drinking."

—The Talmud, 200 B.C.

Swap Out White Wine for Red

Red wine, in moderation, can have quite the positive impact on your health. Studies have shown that red wine may inhibit the formation of fat cells and help prevent obesity by affecting the gene SIRT1. Red wine is also rich in antioxidants that can help raise HDL ("good") cholesterol and protect against heart disease. Its antioxidants come in two forms— flavonoids and nonflavonoids. One of these nonflavonoids is resveratrol, which may help to protect against atherosclerosis and heart disease. It also activates SIRT1, a gene that helps the body process fat, improves overall aerobic activity, and may have a positive impact on longevity.

Alternate Sources

If you don't drink wine, Concord grape juice provides similar nutrients. It is high in polyphenols, which have anti-inflammatory and anti-oxidant properties that help to increase your metabolic rate. A Tufts University study found that Concord grape juice helps increase memory and improve cognitive and motor function as we age. Other studies have shown that the juice helps maintain immune function, and lowers total cholesterol and blood pressure. Remember to keep portions reasonable (4 ounces) to avoid going overboard on calories.

REPLACE RED WINE WITH A BLUEBERRY SMOOTHIE

A report published in the *Journal of Agriculture and Food Chemistry* showed that the blueberry has 38 percent more antioxidants than red wine. One cup of blueberries reportedly provides three to five times the antioxidants found in five servings of carrots, broccoli, squash, and apples. What this means for your health is a lower risk of heart disease; vibrant, firm skin; and a boost in brain power.

"Ballet technique is arbitrary and very difficult.
It never becomes easy; it becomes possible."

—Agnes De Mille

Add Static Balance Poses to Your Workouts

Your body is always looking to find a state of equilibrium. As you age, this process that is controlled by the nervous system begins to slow down. This slowing down process is inevitable, but with training you can prolong the process and live life to the fullest whatever your age.

Practicing balance exercises challenges the nervous system and helps keep the mind-body connection sharp. It also helps to keep the mind and body sharp in the case that balance has to be regained.

Gymnastics, golf, and Tai Chi are all excellent examples of athletic activities that require static balance. Static balance is the type of balance that is most commonly thought of when you think of being able to hold your balance well. This type of balance is exactly what it sounds like—holding a position and not moving. Standing on one leg and holding the other knee up (stork stand) is a static balance exercise.

IT'S A GREAT WAY TO MINIMIZE INJURIES

Balance training is actually a great way to prevent injuries. Static balance exercises are a type of muscular endurance activity. What happens is that in order to hold a position (say on one leg for example), all of the muscles in your foot, knee, and hip are activating. They must activate in order to hold you steady. These muscles are usually the stabilizers that do the work.

Any time you train stabilizing muscles to work you also strengthen connective tissues and joints, and an increase in joint stability and strength equals decreased risk of injury.

"God doesn't make orange juice, God makes oranges."

—Jesse Jackson

Make Vitamin C Consumption a Priority

Vitamin C is a potent antioxidant that is also extremely important for proper brain function and, as such, is found in much higher levels within the brain than other parts of the body. In addition to boosting the effectiveness of other antioxidants, vitamin C is an essential ingredient in the manufacture of several neurotransmitters such as dopamine and acetylcholine. In short, a daily dose of vitamin C can boost and maintain mental acuity. So important is vitamin C to proper brain function that it is being evaluated as a possible nutritional preventative for Alzheimer's disease. Most fruits and vegetables are great sources of vitamin C. Foods particularly high in C include hot chili peppers (raw), cantaloupe, sweet peppers, dark green leafy vegetables, tomatoes, kiwi fruit, oranges, and mango.

Don't Overdo Vitamin C

Because vitamin C is a water-soluble vitamin, your body excretes the excess that may be consumed. Very large doses, though, could cause kidney stones, nausea, and diarrhea. The effects of taking large amounts over extended periods of time are not yet known. You can safely take up to 2,000 milligrams per day (adult), but anything over 2,500 may affect blood or urine tests.

THE WHITE "GREEN" VEGETABLE

The saying "eat your green vegetables" should have the amendment—"and cauliflower." This nutritional powerhouse is a cruciferous vegetable, in the same family as broccoli, cabbage, and kale. It has high levels of vitamin C and significant amounts of vitamin B_6, folate, and dietary fiber.

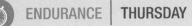
"My heart's in really great shape thanks to spinning classes."

—Christine Lahti

Ramp Up Your Endurance with Spinning Classes

Spinning on a stationary bike is a proven way to reduce body fat and expend calories, but it is much more than that. Spinning also helps you to strengthen joints, lower raised cholesterol, and increase energy levels. In terms of calories burned, about 10 minutes of spinning burns about 115 calories. If you took a spinning class every day over a year for at least 10 minutes a day, it could lead to a 12-pound weight loss. Spinning offers opportunities to strengthen your large leg muscles and increase your workout intensity by adding resistance and speed. Plus, spinning classes will be led by an instructor who will vary the routine from slow to fast, spicing up the session with increased resistance or having you stand as you pedal. A spin class is a quality workout, usually lasting forty-five minutes to an hour.

Plus, training with a group is an excellent way to really enjoy your training. You will often get energy from the group that can make the difference between a poor session and a productive workout. Most cities of reasonable size will have health clubs that offer spinning classes.

If you train frequently with a group, you will learn from the more experienced spinners, and you will learn about new equipment, better nutrition, and different workouts that can add variety to your training. In the end, the top reward for training with others will be the friends you make.

GO FOR THE TOTAL BURN

Some spin classes use stationary bikes that use a flywheel that requires constant pedaling so you can't coast. It's a tough but very effective workout, and you can usually just jump into a spin session at the last minute as long as there is a free bike.

"When you do yoga, the deep breathing, the stretching, the movements that release muscle tension, the relaxed focus on being present in your body . . . the heartbeat slows, respiration decreases, blood pressure decreases. The body seizes this chance to turn on the healing mechanisms."

—Richard Faulds

Flush Out Toxins with Bikram Yoga

Bikram Yoga is a challenging, hot, and aggressive yoga style developed by Bikram Choudhury. The practice consists of a prescribed sequence of twenty-six yoga postures designed to enhance the efficient functioning of every body system. The series is done utilizing the ujjayii breath. The yoga studio is heated up to 100 degrees to encourage sweating and the release of impurities.

Standing postures are done in the first part of the series. Backbends, forward bends, and twists complete the practice along with *kapalabhati breath,* the breath of fire. Each posture is usually performed twice and held for a certain length of time.

People who are already in good shape, with minimal chronic ailments or injuries, are good candidates for Bikram Yoga. It is a practice designed to encourage the cleansing of the body, the releasing of toxins, and maximum flexibility. Bikram Yoga has become increasingly mainstream so you'll likely be able to find a yoga studio that offers classes for you to sample.

YOGA SHOULD NEVER BE PAINFUL

There is a difference between pain and feeling the intensity of an action. Don't force or strain when performing the poses. Strive for a balance between ease and effort. You should feel better after yoga, although some soreness is normal. Soreness is healthy pain, while searing, persistent pain is unhealthy, indicating injury. Injury may require care from a health professional.

"Life is a train of moods like a string of beads; and as we pass through them they prove to be many-colored lenses, which paint the world their own hue, and each shows us only what lies in its own focus."

—Ralph Waldo Emerson

Create Jewelry with Beads

Beading has increased in popularity in recent years and is considered by many to be not only a high art form but also a way to earn some extra bucks. Already, there are several magazines devoted to beading and columns about beading in others. Whether you want to create beaded jewelry or works of art, you'll soon discover that time seems to fly as you discover beads in assorted styles, shapes, colors, and textures; decide on the optimum way to use them; and then create beautiful earrings, chokers, bracelets, pins, and necklaces. To find beads, visit a bead shop, department stores, and arts and crafts outlets. Have fun making your distinctive pieces as gifts for birthdays and other celebratory occasions, showing them in galleries, or selling them in stores or online.

When you learn a new skill, particularly one that involves complex planning and execution, it's particularly good for your brain. If beading or making jewelry is not your cup of tea, choose something that will require new skills, dexterity, and complex thinking—and have fun!

SEARCH THE INTERNET TO FIND LOWER MATERIAL COSTS

Hobbies can be an expensive enterprise. But if you have time and persistence, you can often find items you need for your hobby at competitive prices on the Internet. Teaming up with others who share your interest in a particular hobby can sometimes help you get a better price because you can buy in bulk. Search for those good deals and share them with your friends and colleagues. Buy two for one when possible, such as bags of beads or findings, and look for other ways to reduce your cost of buying hobby materials.

"Who looks outside, dreams; who looks inside, awakes."

—Carl Gustav Jung

Try Reiki to Restore Body and Soul

If you've been feeling particularly stressed, exhausted, and out of whack, treat your body and soul to a Reiki session. Reiki (pronounced ray-key) is an energy healing technique based in ancient Tibetan practices. Practitioners of Reiki put their hands on or just above the body in order to balance energy by acting as a sort of conduit for life force energy. Reiki is used to treat physical problems as well as emotional and psychological problems, and it is, more positively, also used as a tool to support and facilitate positive changes. Becoming a Reiki practitioner is a complex process and also is somewhat mysterious. Advanced Reiki practitioners are even thought to be able to perform long-distance healing.

If you are interested in less mainstream types of massage therapy such as Reiki, but don't know where to find a practioner, talk to friends, a natural health provider, a yoga teacher, or the employees at your local natural health food store for recommendations. Some areas have directories of natural health-care providers.

"By the second tour, I had rice cakes and hummus with me,
and I was jumping rope in my room."

—Taylor Dayne

Eat Hummus

It's hard to complain about hummus. All of the ingredients used to produce it—chickpeas, olive or canola oil, puréed sesame seeds (also known as tahini), lemon juice, spices, and garlic—are extremely good for you and most are known to boost the metabolism. Chickpeas are an excellent source for energy; they're made of complex carbohydrates and protein, and tahini is rich in minerals, fatty acids, and amino acids. So, enjoy, but keep your intake in check because hummus is high in calories; if you're using it as a dip, it's easy to eat a lot of it. It's even better when you spread 2 tablespoons of hummus on a slice of whole-grain bread or eat a ¼ cup of hummus with carrots or broccoli. To make your own hummus try the following recipe.

HUMMUS

1 16-ounce can of chickpeas or garbanzo beans
¼ cup liquid from can of chickpeas
3–5 tablespoons lemon juice (depending on taste)
1½ tablespoons tahini
2 cloves garlic, crushed
½ teaspoon salt
2 tablespoons olive oil

1. Drain chickpeas and set aside liquid from can.
2. Combine remaining ingredients in blender or food processor.
3. Add ¼ cup of liquid from chickpeas.
4. Blend for 3 to 5 minutes on low until thoroughly mixed and smooth. Serve immediately with fresh, warm or toasted pita bread, or cover and refrigerate for up to three days. Add zest by seasoning with red pepper.

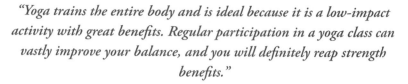

TUESDAY | STRENGTH

"Yoga trains the entire body and is ideal because it is a low-impact activity with great benefits. Regular participation in a yoga class can vastly improve your balance, and you will definitely reap strength benefits."

—Lucia Colbert, triathlon enthusiast

Do the Crescent Pose to Improve Your Static Balance

Static balance poses are similar to what you would see in most Hatha Yoga classes. Here's what you need to know to begin:

- Begin slowly and take as much time as you need to move into a pose or exercise.
- Take your time and be patient. Every small movement or shift of your body weight changes where your center of mass is within the body, and it takes time for the body to adjust to this.
- While working on static balance, fix your gaze on a single spot. At first it should be about one to two feet in front of you and down on the floor.
- As you become more experienced, challenge yourself by bringing your eyes and chin up little by little. The higher your gaze, the more difficult it is to maintain stable balance.
- It is best to practice static balance poses until you can hold them steady for eight to ten seconds. Do each pose one to two times on each side.

The crescent pose is a position that will utilize your legs in very much the same way as a lunge. Your front leg is going to be bent at the knee 90 degrees while your back leg is extended straight out and back like a kickstand. Next, bring your arms up over your head while keeping your rib cage pressed onto the wall of your body. Try to keep your shoulders away from your ears. Take deep, slow breaths in order to stay calm and focused.

"I had a little nut-tree, nothing would it bear;
But a golden nutmeg and a silver pear."

—Mother Goose

Get Plenty of Vitamin E

Vitamin E is an important antioxidant that also restores damaged neurotransmitter receptor sites on neurons. This means that vitamin E both prevents age-related brain deterioration and also reverses a specific aspect of that breakdown. There is also evidence that vitamin E can prevent the onset of Alzheimer's disease and slow its progression once it develops, and that a combination of vitamin E and the mineral selenium can dramatically improve mood and cognitive function in older patients. In addition, vitamin E can help reduce risk of heart disease, stroke, and certain types of cancer. Vitamin E is considered nontoxic, even over RDA (Recommended Daily Allowance) levels. Vitamin E has a UL set at 1,000 mg per day for adults over eighteen. To bolster your vitamin E levels, you can add foods rich in vitamin E, such as dried almonds, vegetable oils, salad dressing, nuts and seeds, wheat germ oil, peanut butter, and green leafy vegetables.

Here's a delicious and nutritious sauce to perk up greens and blanched vegetables. Lemon and parsley nourish liver function to digest fats and oils. Vitamin E and magnesium rich sunflower seeds can support heart and cardiovascular health.

LEMON PARSLEY SUNFLOWER SEED SAUCE

This delicious sauce brightens up greens and blanched vegetables.

Serves 6

½ cup sunflower seeds, toasted

¼ cup olive oil

2 cloves garlic

¾ cup spring water

1 tablespoon lemon juice

2 teaspoons tahini

2 teaspoons umeboshi paste

2 cups parsley, loosely packed

1. Process sunflower seeds in a blender and place in a small bowl. Combine oil, garlic, water, lemon juice, tahini, and umeboshi paste in a blender.
2. Chop parsley finely and add to blender and process. Add sunflower seeds and blend until creamy.

PER SERVING: Calories 170 | **Fat** 16g | **Protein** 3g | **Sodium** 196mg | **Fiber** 2g | **Carbohydrates** 4g

*"I got kicked out of ballet class because
I pulled a groin muscle. It wasn't mine."*

—Rita Rudner

Recharge with an Energy-Boosting Smoothie

The important vitamins, minerals, and antioxidants in this smoothie will provide your body with the boost it needs with a more sustainable effect than the store-bought, chemically enhanced energy drinks.

PINEAPPLE BERRY ENERGY BOOSTER

Recipe Yields: 3–4 cups

1 cup watercress
2 cups pineapple
1 cup strawberries
1 cup blackberries
1 cup purified water

1. Combine watercress, pineapple, strawberries, blackberries, and ½ cup of water in a blender and blend until thoroughly combined.
2. Add remaining ½ cup of water as needed while blending until desired consistency is achieved.

PER 1 CUP SERVING: Calories 65 | **Fat** 0g | **Protein** 1g | **Sodium** 6mg | **Fiber** 3g | **Carbohydrates** 16g

"[Julia] Roberts enjoys a variety of fitness routines that includes swimming, running, cross country skiing, arm exercise, yoga, and Pilates."

—Zeel.com

Cross-Train to Improve Overall Flexibility

Cross-training not only gives you the sustained excitement of different exercises to your mind and body, but also allows you to reap the benefits of every form of exercise. You can strengthen your heart, open your lungs, and build the different muscle types used for quick movements and sustained activity.

To get the most benefit, you should allow your body exposure to different stresses. While any amount of moderate exercise is very beneficial, the most benefit comes from doing different forms of exercises. Serious weight lifters and runners follow this strategy. Weight lifters are always changing their movements and therefore how they stress their muscles. This produces the greatest muscle growth from the constant accommodation to new strains. Runners will vary paces and distances to maximize stress on different types of muscle fibers.

Choose your favorite sports or activities, and divide them up during the week. For example, play racquet ball on Mondays and Friday, take yoga classes on Wednesdays and Sundays; take a long power-walk Monday, Wednesday, and Fridays, and lift weights on Tuesdays and Thursdays. The point is to do things that exercise different parts of your body so muscles are given opportunities to strengthen and joints and ligaments are offered opportunities to limber up and stretch. By cross-training, you'll improve your overall strength and flexibility.

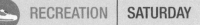

"When your hobbies get in the way of your work—that's OK;
but when your hobbies get in the way of themselves . . . well."

—Steve Martin

Build a Model Airplane, Train, or Ship

As a child, did you ever play with little models of fighter planes and ships or a miniature train set up on tracks with it's own little village? If you did, you probably have some fond memories of that time. There are many advantages to resuming that activity now that you are an adult. For example, you can build a plane, ship, or train alone and enjoy some worry-free downtime. Or, you can spend some quality time working on a favorite model project with a young family member and share with him or her some of the history behind that model. Additionally, if you really get into that hobby, you and your family can visit museums, read books about your models, and plan family vacations to places where that model made history.

Again, if modelmaking doesn't appeal, choose something equally complex, such as knitting or quiltmaking or making stained glass or photography. Make it something that will challenge you, and your brain will thank you for it.

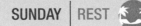
"Now, blessings light on him that first invented sleep! It covers a man all over, thoughts and all, like a cloak; it is meat for the hungry, drink for the thirsty, heat for the cold, and cold for the hot. It is the current coin that purchases all the pleasures of the world cheap, and the balance that sets the king and the shepherd, the fool and the wise man, even."

—Miguel de Cervantes, *Don Quixote*, 1605

Try Hops to Help You Fall Asleep

A thousand years ago brewers of English ale began using hops as a preservative. Science has since recognized the remarkable power of hops as a sedative. It has a calming effect on the body, soothes muscle spasms, relieves nervous tension, and promotes restful sleep. If you suffer from insomnia, make a tea with 1 teaspoon of dried hops in a cup of boiling water and drink it at bedtime. Capsules are also available. Externally, an old-fashioned cure for sleeplessness is to sleep on a small pillowcase filled with hops sprinkled with alcohol.

"A first-rate soup is more creative than a second-rate painting."

—Abraham Maslow

Make It a Green Soup Day

Greens provide amazing health benefits, and one way to maximize their impact is to blend raw greens together to create delicious—and nutritious—juices and soups. Here's a recipe that provides amazing nutrition:

GREEN GAZPACHO

This smoothie is modeled after gazpacho, a delightful cold soup prepared from a tomato base with onions, cucumber, bell pepper, and garlic. It's packed with vitamins and minerals, creating a tasty fiesta in your blender!

Recipe Yields: 3–4 cups
1 cup watercress
2 tomatoes
1 cucumber, peeled
1 celery stalk
½ red onion
½ green pepper
3 garlic cloves
1 small jalapeño (optional)
3 tablespoons red wine vinegar
2 tablespoons basil leaves, chopped
1 cup purified water, if needed

1. Combine all ingredients except the purified water in a blender and blend until thoroughly combined.
2. If needed, slowly add purified water while blending until desired texture is achieved.

PER 1 CUP SERVING: Calories 34 | **Fat** 0g | **Protein** 2g | **Sodium** 18mg | **Fiber** 2g | **Carbohydrates** 7g

"Nothing good comes in life or athletics unless a lot of hard work has preceded the effort. Only temporary success is achieved by taking short cuts."

—Roger Staubach

Do the Warrior III Pose to Improve Static Balance

This pose is done standing on one leg with the opposite leg reaching back behind you. Your arms can be alongside your body, out to the sides, or reaching forward with arms by the ears. At first you may bend the standing leg. Once you have found stability, try to make the standing leg all the way straight. The back leg should reach back vigorously with the foot flexed.

Begin the single-leg standing pose with the knee of one of your legs lifted up in front of you. Your opposite leg, which is going to be your standing/support leg, should be completely straight. Next, take your bent leg and extend it out in front of you as straight and as high as you can. If your standing leg is bending in order to balance you, then you are not ready to hold your leg so high and you will need to lower your extended leg a bit for the moment. As you improve and become more stable in this pose you will be able to lift the extended leg higher. Avoid lifting your extended leg beyond the point where you can maintain balance while keeping both of your legs straight. Bending your knees is just compensating for a lack of strength or flexibility, so it's more important for you to maintain the alignment than to lift the leg as high as possible.

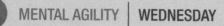

> *"All those vitamins aren't to keep death at bay,*
> *they're to keep deterioration at bay."*
>
> —Jeanne Moreau

Get Plenty of Vitamin B$_{12}$

Vitamin B$_{12}$, produced by intestinal bacteria, is a water-soluble vitamin necessary for proper brain and nerve function, blood formation, and DNA synthesis. An estimated 25 percent of people between ages sixty and seventy are deficient in this essential nutrient, as are nearly 40 percent of people eighty and older. A B$_{12}$ deficiency may be mistaken for an age-related decline in mental function, including memory loss and a reduction in reasoning skills. To hedge your bet, take a multivitamin tablet daily.

Animal products and supplements are the most reliable sources of vitamin B$_{12}$, as miso, storebought tempeh, and sea vegetables contain an analog that is biologically inactive.

FOODS RICH IN VITAMIN B$_{12}$

It's always best to get as many of your vitamins as possible from food sources. These foods are high in vitamin B$_{12}$:

- Liver, beef, lamb
- Crabs, lobster, clams, oysters, and mussels
- Mackerel, herring, salmon, tuna, cod, sardines, trout, and bluefish
- Cheese and eggs

"Excellence is not a singular act, but a habit.
You are what you repeatedly do."

—Shaquille O'Neal

Add Interval Training

An interval is a run of set duration—an hour is typical—with planned increases in speed throughout. For example, on a 400-meter track, you do a warm-up mile (four loops), then pick up your speed to high intensity, but not all out, for two loops or 800 meters. Dial it back down to a jog for the same distance, then do another 800 meters at a hard pace. Or you could kickbox for three minutes, and then do lunges for three minutes; or you jump rope for five minutes and then do bicep curls for five minutes; or run two miles and then walk two; or you run up a set of bleachers and then do a set of yoga stretches before dashing down again.

What is happening with your body in interval training is that in the hard part of the workout, you are in oxygen debt and your body is burning glycogen for fuel. In the recovery part of the workout, your body is making an adaptive response to the workout, creating more capillaries to carry blood (and therefore oxygen) to your system. You are increasing your aerobic capacity and training your body to work hard. It helps give you that extra oomph needed to build endurance.

Some studies have found that interval training alters the mitochondria (the engine-like organelles that produce energy in cells) to burn more fat, which means interval training is a great way to pump up your metabolism and make your workouts more fun.

Your training the day after an interval session should be easy. Complete rest on occasion is advisable.

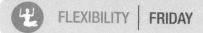

*"Focus on your problem zones, your strength, your energy,
your flexibility and all the rest. Maybe your chest is flabby
or your hips or waist need toning. Also, you should change
your program every thirty days. That's the key."*

—Jack LaLanne

Add Stretch Bands to Your Workouts

Stretch bands come in different styles, some with handles and some without. The bands with handles are the easiest to use. The bands are typically rubber tubing that offer resistance, with handles on each end of the band for ease of use.

The stretch band can also help you with your workouts. One of the best exercises is to hook the band over your feet as you sit on the floor, then pull straight back on the band as though you are rowing. In fact, the exercise is meant to replicate the seated rowing machine you find at health clubs. Be sure to keep your back straight, and when you pull back, make sure your elbows go behind your back.

You can also hang the stretch bands over a door and do "chops," or lat pulls pulling the band downward at an angle. Another option is to attach the band to something on the floor and do your chops in an upward direction. With each stretch band exercise, work up to two sets of twelve repetitions.

"Hobbies of any kind are boring except to people who have the same hobby. This is also true of religion, although you will not find me saying so in print."

—Dave Barry

Join an Association Devoted to Your Hobby

You know you love working on your hobby. Whatever your hobby is, there's undoubtedly a professional association representing it. To find yours, type the name of your hobby into your computer browser and see what it lists. Or, go to *www.hobby.org*, where you will discover the hottest new crafts and hobbies in the global marketplace. For example, scrapbooking, quilting and needlecrafts, art, and framing top the list today. The association(s) for your hobby might host annual competitions, produce a magazine, or provide grants or scholarships so that deserving individuals can learn more about their favorite hobby.

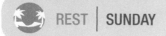
"We make a living by what we do, but we make a life by what we give."

—Winston Churchill

Feed Some Children—Children You Don't Know, but Love

While most of us enjoy some sort of Sunday dinner, children living in Third World countries do not get enough to eat and go without clean drinking water. Create good karma by making a little sacrifice to ensure that a child does not have to endure hunger for another day. Donate a week's worth of money you would spend on going out to eat to *www.feedthechildren.com.*

Other ways you can help include:

- Take a quiz and help end world hunger. Visit *www.worldhunger.org./contributefood.htm* and take the quiz, and Hunger Notes will make a donation to stop world hunger. The undernourished are increasing at the rate of roughly 15 million each year.
- Build your vocabulary and end hunger—at the same time. Visit *www.freerice.com* and play a simple (but addictive) vocabulary game. For every word you get right, the organization donates ten grains of rice through the UN World Food Program.
- Click to Give™ free food. Simply visit *www.thehungersite.com* and click on its homepage—and you've donated one cup of food to the world's hungry. Simple as that.

A QUARTER A DAY MAKES HUNGER GO AWAY

While it might be hard to budget donating large lump sums to organizations, consider setting aside a quarter a day in a hunger fund. Once the quarters start to pile up, take them to the bank and then write out a check (see *www.bread.org* for donating to hunger organizations).

"Taken altogether, the evidence certainly suggests that incorporating at least a few cups of green tea every day will positively affect your health."

—Diane McKay, PhD

Drink Green or Oolong Tea

Green tea has been used as a medicine in China for more than 4,000 years. In the last decade or so, green tea's health benefits have been more widely researched, and many believe the results have shown that it has potential to fight cancer and heart disease. Other studies indicate that it may also help lower cholesterol, burn fat, prevent diabetes and stroke, and hold off dementia.

In addition, green tea and oolong tea contain caffeine and catechins, which have been shown to boost metabolism for approximately two hours. Researchers say drinking 2 to 4 cups of green or oolong tea throughout the day may help you burn an extra 50 calories, which can lead to a five-pound loss over a year—without any other change in your diet. Obviously, adding sugar or cream would counteract the positive effects. Also, avoid green tea beverages that have high-fructose corn syrup, as they are loaded with sugar and are not good for your metabolism.

WEEK FORTY-EIGHT

IT'S GOOD FOR YOUR SKIN TOO!

One of the latest benefits attributed to green tea is that its antioxidants fight against free radicals which damage the skin and prevent cell oxidation and damage that can make you look older than you really are. Studies are mixed on this particular green tea benefit, and some believe you have to apply it topically to experience the full benefits; however, many people have found that potent green tea extracts do have a positive effect on their skin, leaving it softer, more supple, and younger looking.

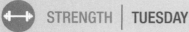

"I do yoga so that I can stay flexible enough
to kick my own arse if necessary."

—Betsy Cañas Garmon, Wildthymecreative.com

Add Dynamic Balance Exercises

Dynamic balance is not only achieved through performing maneuvers with only one support leg, it can also be achieved by practicing and sharpening how you move in a simulated fighting stance. When in this stance, or working on shadowboxing, you may find that it can be easy to lose control of your balance while learning to shift your weight in so many opposing directions. In this case it is also necessary for you to be able to recover your balance in order to keep yourself moving. The ability to keep your COM (see Week Twenty-Four) over your base of support (in this case your feet) will help to maintain balance while moving.

When performing exercises that train dynamic balance, you should perform eight to twelve repetitions and anywhere from one to three sets of each exercise.

Start with Single-Leg Repetition Kicks

While standing on the left leg, bring the right knee forward and up. As the hips move forward, extend the right foot out to complete the kick. Send it out and back in repetition, touching the ball of the foot back on the floor lightly between each kick. Remember, your target is the groin or midsection. This can also be done with a round kick. Turn the base foot out, lift the kicking leg knee up, and extend the kick out and back and again lightly touch the foot to the floor between each kick. Be sure you recoil the kick as this will help you stay balanced. The target for a round kick is the rib cage.

When performing exercises that train dynamic balance, you should perform eight to twelve repetitions and anywhere from one to three sets of each exercise.

"In the beginner's mind there are many possibilities,
in the expert's mind there are few."

—Shunryu Suzuki, *Zen Mind, Beginner's Mind*

Be as Receptive as a Baby

According to Alison Gopnik, author of *The Philosophical Baby: What Children's Minds Tell Us About Truth, Love, and the Meaning of Life*, babies have the ultimate "beginner's mind." A beginner's mind is one that embraces an attitude of openness, eagerness, and lack of preconceptions when studying a subject. It is highly prized in Zen Buddhism and Japanese martial arts.

As we grow up, our brain undergoes a pruning process that narrows our perception of life, which can lead to limited creativity and decreased ability to problem solve. This pruning also limits our ability to "be in the now," and leaves us less open and less flexible. A baby's brain, on the other hand, has more brain cells and fewer inhibitory neurotransmitters than adults. Their brains have an amazing, almost supersonic ability to sort through lots of excess information and remain more receptive to discovering highly rewarding solutions or intriguing, innovative concepts. A baby's brain notices the beauty and wonder around it and lives, very much, "in the now."

You may not be able to completely recapture a baby's state of mind, but you can consciously choose to live mindfully, in the now, looking at new experiences and new people with a fresh eye. In other words, learn to tamp down your inhibitors, observe without judgment, and gather as much unbiased information as possible before allowing your more "mature" mind to make its usual assumptions or respond in your typical fashion.

"It's a great art, is rowing. It's the finest art there is. It's a symphony of motion. And when you're rowing well it's nearing perfection. And when you reach perfection, you're touching the divine. It touches the you of you's, which is your soul."

—George Pocock

Join a Rowing Club

Rowing exercises larger muscle groups in both the upper and lower body. It is, in fact, one of the best forms of total body aerobic exercise because it involves all the major muscle groups. Also, within ten minutes of rowing, your body gets into a rhythm that lights your metabolic fire. Rowing tones the arms and builds upper-body strength. Rowing for twenty-five minutes is aerobically equal to forty minutes on a stationary bike. In a kayak or rowboat, you can get a workout targeting the core areas of your body, but if you like working out with others, join a rowing club.

Basically, rowing takes two forms. When rowers have an oar in each hand, it's called sculling. When rowers have both hands on one oar, it is called sweep rowing. Rowing is a low-impact exercise but does require a degree of agility, grace, and teamwork. Rowing as a team teaches you to work together for maximum effectiveness. The boat advances more rapidly when the team members row quickly and in unison. So make some new friends, learn the art of rowing, get in a regular workout, and feel good as your body becomes trim and toned—and your metabolism ratchets up.

"I love to ride my bike, which is great aerobics, but also just a great time for me to think, so it's like this terrific double bill."

—Robin Williams

Make Sure You Include Aerobic Exercise

Aerobic exercise provides a wealth of benefits. Even if you don't need to tone up or lose weight, it's great for you. Each week, aim for at least 150 minutes of moderate-intensity exercise (this means you can talk but can't sing, or if you're using a heart rate monitor, it is 55–69 percent of your maximum heart rate) for at least twenty minutes at a time. This will get your heart rate/circulation up and improve the oxygen flow to your body, which, in turn, will help boost your metabolism.

If you're looking for other reasons to inspire you to exercise, here are just a few:

- Exercising regularly reduces your risk of heart disease, type II diabetes, stroke, certain types of cancer, and osteoporosis.
- Exercising regularly and burning at least 800 calories per week could have a beneficial impact on your cholesterol by raising your HDL (the "good cholesterol") and lowering your LDL (the "bad cholesterol") and triglycerides.
- Aerobic exercise reduces muscle tension and the amount of stress hormones in your body so you'll feel less wound up during the day and sleep better at night.
- Aerobic exercise boosts endorphins—even before you reach that "runner's high"—and releases additional serotonin in your brain, which helps to balance your mood or relieve depression.
- Exercising improves circulation, which not only flushes away harmful toxins that can damage your skin but also protects against fine lines and wrinkles.

"Volunteers do not necessarily have the time;
they just have the heart."

—Elizabeth Andrew

Volunteer Your Time

Rather than spend your Saturdays running errands, how about volunteering to help out at your local hospital. Variously called Candy Stripers and Pink Ladies, these volunteers (men are included, too) serve an important function in hospitals that are often understaffed. Volunteers can rock babies to sleep, operate the hospitality cart offering magazines and gum, fetch wheelchairs, and transport discharged patients to their cars. You'll help out and get exercise, as well.

Other ways to volunteer your time include:

- Read to the blind. You can help record audio versions of newspapers, books, and magazines for the visually impaired. Check out Learning Ally (*www.learningally.org*) today and volunteer.
- Become a Red Cross volunteer. The Red Cross is perhaps the best-known relief organization offering medical and other types of help in times of disaster. See *www.redcross.org* for more information.

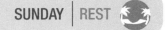
"Soon silence will have passed into legend. Man has turned his back on silence. Day after day he invents machines and devices that increase noise and distract humanity from the essence of life, contemplation, meditation . . . tooting, howling, screeching, booming, crashing, whistling, grinding, and trilling bolster his ego. His anxiety subsides. His inhuman void spreads monstrously like a gray vegetation."

—Jean Arp

Turn Down the Noise

If you always have to have the television or the radio on, whether you are watching it or not, if you can't get yourself to work or do your homework without music or television in the background (or foreground), if you've tried to meditate but absolutely can't stand the silence, if you always fall asleep to the television or to music, then you've probably got a noise habit.

Silence can be not only therapeutic but also remarkably energizing. Finding a space each day for silence and stillness allows the body to recharge. There is nothing wrong with noise, but constant noise keeps your mind from focusing completely on anything and encourages fragmentation. You may be able to get your work or your homework done in front of the television, but it will probably take you longer and you probably won't do as good a job.

People who live alone often like to keep noise in the background. Noise can temporarily mask your loneliness or nervousness. It can calm an anxious mind or distract a troubled mind. Constant noise can provide a welcome relief from oneself, but if it is compromising your ability to think and perform as well as you could, if it is keeping you from confronting your stress and yourself, then it's time to make some space for silence in your life. Too much noise is stressful on the body and the mind. Give yourself a break and let yourself experience silence at least once each day for at least ten minutes. Don't be afraid of silence. To quote Martha Stewart, "It's a good thing."

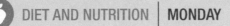

*"It's difficult to think anything but pleasant thoughts
while eating a homegrown tomato."*

—Lewis Grizzard

Eat Vibrantly Colored Vegetables

The more colors on the plate, the more health-promoting properties there are as well. The colors in vegetables give hints about their vitamin content. Dark leafy greens are high in B vitamins, while red and yellow vegetables are good sources of vitamins A and C. Eating a wide variety of different colored vegetables ensures a broad spectrum of essential vitamins. About 25–30 percent of the weight of your daily food intake should be bright, vibrant vegetables.

"We don't know who we are until we see what we can do."

—Martha Grimes

Add a Front Kick–Back Kick Combination

Another great dynamic balance exercise (see Week Forty-Five) is a front kick–back kick combination. Remember that it's important to keep your COM (center of mass), generally just below your navel and in an inch over your base of support to maintain balance in any movement.

Send a left leg front kick, place the foot down underneath you, and immediately send a right leg back kick. In order to perform a back kick, you lift the knee of the kicking leg—in this case it will be the right leg—then extend the leg out behind you. As you kick, think about making contact with the heel of the foot and the toes pointed toward the floor. Recoil the kick and repeat.

The emphasis here is to work on shifting the hips forward and back into each kick. You may look behind you as you send the back kick, but it is not necessary for this particular drill. Looking forward and back in repetition can make anyone dizzy, and that's not the best thing for balance.

When performing exercises that train dynamic balance, you should perform eight to twelve repetitions and anywhere from one to three sets of each exercise.

"The United States ranks first among countries in soft drink consumption. The per-capita consumption of soft drinks is in excess of 150 quarts per year, or about three quarts per week."

—Michael Murray, ND and Joseph Pizzorno, ND,
Encyclopedia of Natural Medicine

"Just Say No" to Soda

The brain uses 65 percent of the body's glucose, but too much or too little glucose can have a detrimental effect on brain function. When you drink a can of soda, which contains 10 teaspoons of table sugar, that sugar is absorbed into a bloodstream that only contains a total of 4 teaspoons of blood sugar. The blood sugar level rockets to an excessive level, setting off alarms in the pancreas, and a large amount of insulin comes out to deal with the excess blood sugar. Some sugar is quickly ushered into the cells, including brain cells, and the rest is put into storage or into fat cells. When all this is done, maybe in about one hour, the blood sugar may fall dramatically and low blood sugar occurs. These rapid swings in blood sugar produce symptoms of impaired memory and clouded thinking.

PLUG UP BRAIN DRAINS

Alcohol, sugar, aspartame sweetener, and MSG all interfere with brain function. Alcohol makes you dull; sugar makes you foggy; aspartame and MSG are brain excitotoxins and can lead to brain cell death.

"Stadiums are for spectators.
We runners have nature and that is much better."

—Juha Vaatainen

Take a Running Vacation

The folks at *Runner's World* decided to rate the twenty-five best cities for running in the United States. How did they do it? According to them, they "tabulated the number of running clubs and races in the largest U.S. cities . . . how much park area is available in each city for runners, how average precipitation levels and temps compared to the competition, and even how crime rates stacked up . . . ." Their system is quite impressive and is detailed on their website at *www.runnersworld.com* under "The 25 Best Running Cities." Their annotated list provides runners with a "must run," a favorite race, a celebrated place to eat, and where to get help in that city. Here's their list of the Top 25:

1. San Francisco, California
2. San Diego, California
3. New York City, New York
4. Chicago, Illinois
5. Washington, D.C.
6. Minneapolis/St. Paul, Minnesota
7. Boulder, Colorado
8. Boston, Massachusetts
9. Denver, Colorado
10. Portland, Oregon
11. Austin, Texas
12. Seattle, Washington
13. Philadelphia, Pennsylvania
14. Colorado Springs, Colorado
15. Dallas, Texas
16. Anchorage, Alaska
17. Raleigh, North Carolina
18. Salt Lake City, Utah
19. Honolulu, Hawaii
20. Atlanta, Georgia
21. Houston, Texas
22. Phoenix, Arizona
23. Madison, Wisconsin
24. Monterey, California
25. Fort Collins, Colorado

"Your body can only tolerate being in one position for about 20 minutes before it starts to feel uncomfortable. About every 15 minutes, stand, stretch, walk around or change your position for at least 30 seconds."

—The Mayo Clinic

Take Time to Stretch at Work

Sitting at a desk all day is hard on your body, and remembering to stretch your muscles occasionally can improve your flexibility—and your attitude. You only need a minute or two of stretching to feel great. First, while sitting on a chair, put both feet on the floor, drop your shoulders away from your ears, and put your hands on your thighs. Take a few deep breaths, as slow as you can. Now, gently drop your head forward (don't force it) and hold for a few seconds. Now, roll your head to the right, chin toward your shoulder. Hold, roll your head back to center, and then roll your head to the left.

Keeping your shoulders down, bring your arms in front of your chest, clasp your fingers, and reach your arms forward, stretching your back. Now stand up, put your hands on your lower back, and press your pelvis forward, leaning your upper body back. Bring your arms behind you and stretch your chest. If you can, bring one knee at a time up to your chest, then reverse that stretch and bring your heel to your butt, holding it with your hand. Go back to your day!

HOW TO REJUVENATE YOURSELF DURING A MEETING

We all get stressed or occasionally bored in meetings that drag on and on. While stretching might call too much attention to yourself, you can rejuvenate your energy by deep breathing. Without closing your eyes, start to focus on deepening the length of your inhales and exhales and, as you do this, focus on bringing your breath to each tense part of your body. This should relax you (on the exhale) and, at the same time, energize you (on the inhale).

"If adventure has a final and all-embracing motive, it is surely this: we go out because it is our nature to go out, to climb mountains, and to paddle rivers, to fly to the planets and plunge into the depths of the oceans. . . . When man ceases to do these things, he is no longer man."

—Wilfrid Noyce

Trek the Himalayas

If you've ever wanted to break out of the ordinary routine and taste adventure, trekking might be just the thing to try. Trekking regions of the Himalayas used to be only for adventurers, mountain climbers, and tourists with a liking for remote and exotic destinations. Today, trekking has become a popular pastime for ordinary people with a chunk of time and enough money to get to Nepal or India. It's a good idea for you to join a trekking group if you are a first-time trekker. Trekking, defined generally as walking while carrying a backpack, will take you through lots of different types of terrain if you are walking in regions of the Himalayas. As you hike, you'll burn lots of calories. Your muscles will become firmer and stronger and you'll begin to feel mental, spiritual, and physical renewal. Read up on trekking; give it a try.

Incidentally, you don't have to go all the way to the Himalayas. You can find trekking opportunities everywhere. Go online and find areas near you just waiting for you to explore.

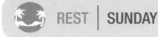

"I think a lot of contemplation happens in bathtubs.
It does for me. Nothing like a hot bath to ease the
tension and think about what's going to happen next."

—Sarah McLachlan

Try a Body Scan to Release Tension

The body scan is a popular relaxation technique that involves a mental scanning of your entire body in search of tension, followed by the conscious release of that tension. You can do a body scan on your own, or you can have someone direct you by speaking out loud and naming the parts of the body, in order (head, forehead, face, neck, jaw, throat, chest, arms, hands, and so on), so that you are cued when to relax what. You can also recite your own body scan cues onto a tape or digital file and play it back for yourself.

Different people do the body scan in different ways. Some people like to tense each area of the body in turn, and then fully relax it. Others prefer to visualize the release of tension without actually contracting the muscles first. You can imagine breathing into and out of each body part, exhaling the tension one area at a time. Whichever way you choose is fine. You might try several ways to find out which one you prefer.

The body scan is a great way to wind down after work or to calm down before a stressful event. Practiced every day, it can become a way to maintain a tension-free body and a body-aware mind. All you need is a quiet place to lie down . . . in fact, this is a great way to relax before bedtime.

"The thing about the Japanese diet is, you don't have to do it every meal. Just incorporate it little by little and see how you feel. By eating more modest portions, more vegetables, less bad fat and drinking green tea instead of soda and eating brown rice, all these little things add up to a very healthy way to eat."

—Naomi Moriyama

Make Brown Rice Your Friend

Brown rice contains far more soluble fiber (preceded only by oats and barley) than traditional white rice, and thus is far better for your health. Here's a saucy recipe that will help you fall in love with brown rice:

BROWN RICE NUT PILAF

Add this pilaf to roasted squash, dolmas, or cabbage rolls. Sauté ½ cup diced carrots, ½ cup diced celery, and ½ cup diced onion in oil until cooked through. Mix sautéed vegetables and ¼ cup toasted walnuts with 2 cups cooked red japonica and brown rice. Season the pilaf with umeboshi vinegar, toasted sesame oil, tahini or hummus, and nori.

1. Preheat oven to 400°F. Line a sheet pan with parchment paper. Cut squash in half lengthwise and scoop out seeds and pulp. Combine oil, salt, and spices together in a small bowl. Brush squash with spice mixture. Arrange cut-side down on prepared baking sheet. Roast for 45–50 minutes or until tender.
2. Mix currants or dried cranberries into Brown Rice Nut Pilaf. Fill each squash with grains.

"I was captain and should have set the example. I would lift a minimum of weights. Mine was natural physical strength. I always thought quickness and agility were much more important."

—Merlin Olsen

Work on Your Agility

The standard definition of agility is the ability to change directions quickly. Most sports require players to stop and start their movements at the drop of a hat. Even dancers must train for agility. In soccer, for example, players run up and down the field with little to no rest throughout the game. They could be running in one direction and in an instant have to decelerate, stabilize the momentum of their bodyweight, coordinate the shift of that weight, create enough momentum to start moving that weight in a new direction, and accelerate as quickly as possible. This is why agility is dependent on strength, speed, coordination, and dynamic balance. If you can train for all of these elements, you will experience an improvement in your agility. The more you practice agility, and the components found within agility, the more your agility will improve.

You will grow stronger through strength and functional training exercises, faster through the practice of speed training and speed drills, more coordinated through functional training exercises where the limbs have to move correctly with each other, and create a better center of balance through the practice of balancing drills, all the while becoming a more well-rounded athlete.

*"Give me golf clubs, fresh air, and a beautiful partner,
and you can keep the clubs and the fresh air."*

—Jack Benny

Join a Social Club

According to researchers, the more people participate in close social relationships, the better their overall physical and mental health, and the higher their level of function. The definition of social relationship is broad and can include everything from daily phone chats with family to regular visits with close friends to attending church every Sunday.

The MacArthur Foundation Study on Aging revealed that the two strongest predictors of well-being among the elderly are frequency of visits with friends and frequency of attendance at organization meetings. And the more meaningful the contribution in a particular activity, the greater the health benefit. And it doesn't always have to be people who believe what you believe. Studies show that the more diverse our innermost circle of social support, the better off we are.

Start Your Own Club

If you can't find a social club you want to join, consider starting your own. Pick something that offers exercise—physical or mental—and you double the benefit. Here are a few ideas:

- Choose activities that involve learning totally new skills, such as sculpting, photographing nature, printmaking, jewelry making, knitting, golfing, or woodworking.
- Choose activities that will require you to think or strategize, such as playing chess, having bunco parties, hosting book clubs, or attending lectures on neuroscience.

The point is to interact regularly with people who stimulate your mind and to be with people who support your quest to learn or improve.

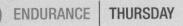

"Camaraderie is one of the main benefits of joining a running club. It gives you the opportunity to socialize and meet other runners. You exchange information, pick up running tips, maybe even find a training partner."

—Linda Hyer, former president of a New Jersey running club

Join a Running Club

There are a number of excellent running clubs around the world that are easy to find, inexpensive to join, and that sponsor activities you can participate in on either a particular weekend or all year. Belonging to a running club is a good way to stay motivated, learn from others, meet people with similar interests, and participate in challenging events. Some clubs are big—like those associated with well-known marathons such as the Boston Athletic Club and the New York Road Runners' Club. Sparsely populated areas have smaller clubs. Different clubs have different personalities.

In the United States, the best place to start is with the granddaddy of them all, the Road Runners' Club of America (RRCA) at *www.rrca.org*. Not only can you find local and national club listings through the RRCA, you can get an idea of what's happening with running across the country. To find clubs in the state where you live or a state you're planning to visit, you can go straight to a map on their website, click on the state, and immediately access a list of all the running clubs in that state. The RRCA's full contact information is as follows:

RRCA National Office

Phone: (703) 525-3890

www.rrca.org

"Climbing to the top demands strength, whether it is to the top of Mount Everest or to the top of your career."

—Abdul Kalam, Indian Statesman

Go Climb a Wall . . . Really

Climbing walls are appearing in more and more gyms, community centers, and schools. Not only is it fun, climbing provides an excellent total-body workout and is mentally and physically challenging, combining balance with footwork and technique. Gyms with indoor climbing walls have the ropes and equipment you need on hand, so you don't have to invest in them. Although it doesn't give a high-intensity cardiovascular workout, it's another way to stretch your muscles while challenging yourself—and can be very entertaining.

WARM UP WITH A WALK

A relaxed 2–3 mile stroll is a great way to loosen up your legs and prepare them for the climb. It will warm up your muscles and get the fluid moving in your joints, readying them for unusual stretches or positions.

"The ultimate aim of Karate lies not in victory or defeat but in the perfection of the character of its participants."

—Gichin Funakoshi

Take a Kickboxing Class

Release some of that aggression in a kickboxing class where you'll learn to combine martial arts kicks with boxing punches for a great workout. Learning to jab, uppercut, roundhouse, and more is sure to boost your self-esteem and confidence, plus it will give you some self-defense skills and melt away those pounds. You'll be working your entire body intensely for forty-five minutes to an hour in an interval-style workout that will burn calories with cardio and require you to engage in strength-training moves that will tone your arms, legs, core, and butt. Stressed about your job or anything else in your life? This is a great, positive place to let all of that anger out.

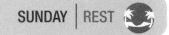

"The mantra becomes one's staff of life and carries one through every ordeal. Each repetition has a new meaning, carrying you nearer and nearer to God."

—Mahatma Ghandi

Try a Mantra Meditation

Mantra meditation is an ancient tradition practiced by many different cultures in many ways. If time is the ultimate test, then mantra meditation may be the ultimate form of meditation. It disciplines the mind, hones the focus, and even improves the depth of the breath and the capacity of the lungs. It's also supremely relaxing.

Concentrated focusing while repeating a sound can be called a mantra meditation, whether it's Sufi chanting or the recitation of the rosary prayer. Some people believe that the sounds of a mantra actually contain certain powers; others believe that the key to mantra meditation is not the sound but the repetition itself. In either case, if you choose a word that means something to you, you may feel your meditation has a more personalized meaning and feeling to it. Any word or phrase will do. Here are a few you might try (the possibilities, of course, are endless):

- Peace
- Love
- Goddess
- Mind, body, spirit
- Hallelujah
- I am happy (or good or special or loving)
- Amen
- Shalom

"The only way to keep your health is to eat what you don't want, drink what you don't like, and do what you'd rather not."

—Mark Twain

Eat Foods Rich in Iron

Almost two-thirds of the iron in your body is found in hemoglobin, the protein in red blood cells that carries oxygen to your body's tissues. Smaller amounts are found in myoglobin, a protein that helps supply oxygen to muscle. About 15 percent of your body's iron is stored for future needs and activated when dietary intake is inadequate. Iron is also needed for a strong immune system and for energy production. In the United States, iron deficiency is one of the most common nutrient deficiencies. Iron deficiency can lead to anemia, fatigue, and infections.

Foods rich in iron include beef liver, fortified cereals, lean red meats, nuts, seeds, poultry, bran, spinach, salmon, legumes, lentils, whole-wheat bread, and wheat germ. It is best to seek the advice of your doctor before taking an iron supplement.

Don't Overdo Iron

Iron supplementation may be indicated when an iron deficiency is diagnosed and when diet alone cannot restore bodily iron content to normal levels within an acceptable time frame. Taking iron supplements can cause side effects such as nausea, vomiting, constipation, diarrhea, dark-colored stools, and abdominal distress. To minimize these side effects, take only what your doctor recommends and take the supplement in divided doses and with food.

"Studies show that regular physical activity combined with good nutrition is the most effective method to ensure long-term weight management."

—Shirley S. Archer, fitness professional,
Stanford University School of Medicine

Spice Up Your Workouts

Variety is the spice of exercise. No matter what types of exercise you choose, you'll work a wider range of muscles and reap a wider range of benefits if you vary your exercise. Try a different kind of activity once a week.

Also, varying your pace can add up to increased health benefits. Author and exercise physiologist Greg Landry, MS, suggests interval training, a simple way to vary any exercise you're already doing. Landry suggests warming up for five minutes, then exercising at your regular pace for four minutes, then stepping up the pace for one minute. Then, for the rest of your workout, work four minutes at a regular pace, then one minute at a fast pace, and so forth. Interval training can help you to break past a weight loss plateau, help get you in shape faster, increase your energy and your body's rate of calorie burning by raising your base metabolism rate, and keep your workout more interesting. Changing pace every five minutes may also help to keep you more focused on your workout, too, which is a nice break for your busy brain.

"Stress is nothing more than a socially accepted mental illness."

—Richard Carlson

Curb Your Stress

An October 2000 *Brain Research Bulletin* study confirmed what has been known since the mid-1980s: Cortisol levels are high in Alzheimer's patients. This study also showed that high levels of cortisol correlated with a more rapid deterioration of the Mini-Mental State Examination (a 30-point questionnaire used to screen for dementia) over a forty-month period in a group of elderly women. Chronic stress elevates cortisol levels, which is one of the main causes of brain cell death.

Stress is also one of the most common causes of transient insomnia; it keeps the brain awake and functioning long into the night or wee hours of the morning. Stress causes worry, and worry interferes with sleep. Excessive stress creates tension and anxiety and can lead to a variety of health problems that are not obviously linked to tension. Stress can also complicate pre-existing conditions.

These are the key symptoms of stress:

- Inability to relax
- Emotional instability/mood swings
- Headaches
- Sleeplessness

Popular stress reduction techniques include regular prayer, meditation, and self-hypnosis. Exercise is also a great way to reduce stress. If chronic stress continues, narrow down its causes and make changes in your life that will bring your stress level down.

"Anyone can run twenty miles. It's the next six that count."

—Barry Magee

Create Your Own Mini-Triathlon

One reason that coaches urge athletes, especially runners, to cross-train is that it saves wear and tear on the body. Swimming, in fact, is an ideal cross-training activity because you don't experience the pounding that you do when you run, but you still get a very useful cardiovascular workout as you make your way back and forth in the pool. You will probably find when you jump into the pool for the first time that there is nothing easy about negotiating the 50 meters down and back in the pool, but it won't give you shin splints or runner's knee. Similarly, biking also provides a good workout for your heart and lungs without beating up your legs.

So why not create your own triathlon by doing all three sports in one day? Each activity offers you opportunities to deepen your workouts, by perfecting your stride as you run, keeping low on your bicycle to decrease wind resistance, and learning long, slow strokes as you swim.

Start slowly, taking breaks between each activity, but as your strength and endurance increase, take shorter and shorter breaks. If you're lucky enough to have a swimming pool, you can shorten transition times even more. If you don't own a pool, you can still intensify your workouts and gain maximum benefit by increasing the length of time you spend on each, or the speed with which you perform.

THREE SPORTS IN ONE

Do not think of a triathlon as three individual sports—swimming, cycling, and running. A triathlon is one sport with three separate phases. You don't get credit for any of them unless you complete all three—even when you're doing them just for fun, to increase your overall endurance.

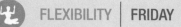

"At times of great stress it is especially necessary to achieve a complete freeing of the muscles."

—Konstantin Stanislavsky

Use Exercise Bands to Stretch Your Shoulders at Work

If you're someone who sits hunched over a desk for six to ten hours a day, you really need to add shoulder stretches to your daily routine. Slumping over a desk causes tightness in your back, neck, and shoulders, which can lead to increased pain and headaches. Luckily, you can do these simple stretches at your desk. All you need is a rubber stretch band that will offer moderate resistance.

While seated at your desk, push back slightly, lay the resistance band on your lap, grip both ends, straighten your spine, lifting your head slightly, and then slowly raise the band up over your head. Once the band is above your head, slowly spread your shoulders, using the resistance in the band to move your shoulder muscles slightly backward. Hold for ten to thirty seconds, pause to breathe deeply, then stretch three more times.

ADD YOGA POSTURES

It's also very helpful to add a few yoga poses to your stretching session. Some that will offer relief to your lower back are reclining child's pose (see Week Twenty-Five), legs up the wall (see Week Thirty-Six), and downward facing dog (see Week Thirty-Seven).

"Whoever said money can't buy happiness simply
didn't know where to go shopping."

—Bo Derek

Shop with a Cause

If shopping online is something you consider recreation, did you know that you could shop certain sites and give to charity at the same time? Purchase items in the "hunger site store," "child health site store," "literacy site store," "rainforest site store," and "animal rescue site store." See *www.greatergood.com* for more information.

Other ways to use your purchasing power to support worthwhile causes include:

- Sponsor a woman. The organization Women for Women (*www .womenforwomen.org*) helps women in war-ravaged countries such as Afghanistan and Rwanda to rebuild their lives. Visit the site to learn about sponsorship, volunteering, and getting involved. You can also send a message of support or shop the bazaar.
- Give fair trade presents. Next time you need a birthday, holiday, or "just because" present, skip the obvious and head for a store where you'll find unique items that also do good internationally. At stores like Ten Thousand Villages (*www.tenthousandvillages .com)* you'll find lots of fair trade goodies that will make the perfect gift.
- Raise awareness while you charge. If you bank with Bank of America and want to make a difference the next time you use your credit card, sign up for its My Expression banking program. Your new credit card will help the cause of your choice.

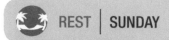

"If you want to lift yourself up, lift up someone else."

—Booker T. Washington

Spend the Day Helping Someone Who Is Sick

Sundays are a perfect day for doing something for others. Here are three ways you can do something that can make a big difference to someone who is sick.

- Make a prayer quilt for a sick person. It takes only two yards of material (soft colors with peaceful images), washed, ironed, and sewn together. The only requirement is that you must pray for healing for the person who will receive the quilt. Pray before starting the quilt and during every step of making it. Singing hymns is considered acceptable as prayer. Have a priest, minister, or congregation bless the quilt before it goes to a hospital patient or a shut-in.
- Make tiny hats for preemies. Donate these knitted caps to your local hospital or a family you know who's recently had a premature baby. Make the hats from washed and dried soft cotton. Call the hospital neonatal unit to find out if they have rules or criteria for making such items.
- Volunteer at a local hospice organization. You will be supporting someone through the process of dying. Each person has to go through the stages of dying alone albeit often surrounded by family, friends, and a support team that will include a hospice nurse and doctor. A patient who is terminal has the right to use his own powers of reason and choice about his care and options as he lives each moment until death occurs. Find out more at *www.hospicenet.org*.

"We are living in a world today where lemonade is made from artificial flavors and furniture polish is made from real lemons."

—Alfred E. Newman

Use Herbs Liberally

Herbs are a great way to add fresh taste and aroma to food, and many provide vitamins and minerals essential to your body's overall health. Here is a list of some herbs and the benefits they provide:

- Basil provides vitamins C and A, plus beta-carotene.
- Chives provide calcium, phosphorous, and several vitamins.
- Cilantro is renowned for its anti-cholesterol, anti-diabetic, and anti-inflammatory effects.
- Dill is rich in antioxidants and dietary fibers that help control blood cholesterol levels.
- Mint, including peppermint and spearmint, has the ability to cut off the blood supply to cancer tumors.
- Oregano is among the best sources of vitamin K, and it has anti-oxidants that prevent cellular damage caused by oxidation of free radicals.
- Rosemary provides carnosic acid, which shields the brain from free radicals and lowers the risk of stroke and neurodegenerative diseases.
- Tarragon is packed with minerals and vitamins C, B_6, A, and E, and may help transfer nutrients to your muscles.

WEEK FIFTY-TWO

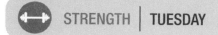

"The dancer's body is simply the luminous manifestation of the soul."

—Isadora Duncan

Dance to Strengthen Your Muscles

As we've mentioned several times, dancing is a marvelous exercise. It's great for your flexibility, but it's also a way to strengthen your muscles. Here's a rundown of the calories you'll burn and the muscles each type of dance strengthens.

- Ballroom dancing: Burns 150 calories an hour. Strengthens leg, shoulder, ab, arm, back, and glute muscles; increases flexibility; improves concentration; only increases heart strength if you do fast steps, such as swing dancing.
- Ballet: Burns 150 calories per hour. Strengthens leg, shoulder, ab, arm, back, and glute muscles; increases flexibility; does not increase cardio power (you need concentration and stamina).
- Country line dancing: Burns 125 calories an hour. Strengthens leg, shoulder, ab, arm, back, and glute muscles.
- Disco dancing: Burns 175 calories an hour. Strengthens leg, shoulder, ab, arm, back, and glute muscles; strengthens the heart.
- Salsa dancing: Burns 170 calories an hour. Strengthens leg, shoulder, ab, arm, back, and glute muscles; increases flexibility and strengthens the heart.

"Silence is the source of great strength."

—Lao Tzu

Improve Your Memory by Turning Down the Noise

The most striking area in which older people and younger people differ is in how they remember. In general, younger people are more adept at learning and retaining information in the face of distractions such as television, loud music, or crowds. Their brains, it seems, are better at multitasking, that is, engaging in several functions at once, such as watching a movie on TV while cramming for a history exam. Older people, as a rule, require a quieter environment in which to digest new information for later retrieval. Studies have concluded that this dramatic generational difference in learning and memorizing is due to the fact that older people have greater difficulty filtering out useless stimuli, such as music or conversation. Their brains absorb everything, affecting the memorization of pertinent information. For this reason, seniors are encouraged to read or study in a quiet environment, where they won't be easily distracted and can focus on the task at hand. Silence can be not only therapeutic but also remarkably energizing. Finding a space each day for silence and stillness allows the body to recharge.

"One way to loosen up the entire body is to go for a light swim. The water is naturally relaxing and will help lessen the tension in all of your muscles. A yoga class can also promote flexibility and relaxation."

—Lucia Colbert, triathlon enthusiast

Opt for Low-Level Activities after Hard Workouts

You may feel great after a workout as the endorphins kick in, and you can't wait for the next training session. Do yourself a favor. Wait. After a particularly demanding workout, rest is how your body grows stronger. It uses the downtime to rebuild from the stresses of your training.

If you follow one hard workout with another, your body will not have a chance to rebuild damaged tissue. Eventually, it will start breaking down rather than regenerating. The bottom line will be injury. You may have to force yourself to go easy the day after an excellent workout, but common sense must rule or you will find yourself in trouble.

One of the by-products of physical activity is lactic acid, which builds up in the muscles during vigorous exercise. When you feel a burning sensation in your calf muscles and thighs, that's lactic acid. Some of it will be removed naturally, but it can build up. As you train, you will increase what is known as your lactate threshold, the point at which your body can no longer remove lactic acid on its own. The higher the threshold, the more you can work at high intensity without feeling the effects of lactic acid in your system.

You can engage in "active rest" the day after a vigorous workout. A typical active rest session would be an easy bike ride or a swim at low to moderate intensity. An easy swim helps remove lactic acid that has accumulated.

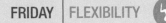

"I feel a lot healthier when I'm having sex. Physically. I feel all these jitters when I wake up in the morning. Just energy jitters. I take vitamins, I work out every day. When I'm having sex, I don't have that."

—Alyssa Milano

Have More Sex

Sex is not only fun, it's also a great way to keep your body limber and healthy. In case you've been going through a long, dry spell, here are five more reasons to have more sex:

1. The more sex you have, the more your brain links the physical closeness of your partner to feelings of trust, empathy, and generosity. It's why sex is so important in marriage and why sexless marriages tend to fall apart at some point.
2. Having sex releases oxytocin, a neuromodulator that sensitizes your body's response to endorphins, which often act as natural painkillers, particularly for headaches. Yes, that's right, having sex can *cure* headaches.
3. Having sex increases blood circulation, which pumps oxygen to your brain—and to your skin—creating the highly desirable post-coital glow.
4. The more sex you have on a regular basis, the more your blood circulation improves, which helps keep your body healthy and functioning overall, and keeps you youthful.
5. Sex boosts your natural collagen production, which minimizes age spots and sagging.
6. Having an orgasm has been shown to decrease chronic pain by 50 percent, and having sex three times a week has been shown to decrease the chance of heart attack and stroke by 50 percent, especially in women.

"Every once in a while, a girl has to indulge herself."

—Sarah Jessica Parker

Take a Spa Day

Save up for a spa day. For both men and women, the experience of pampering yourself at a luxurious spa can be a very relaxing experience as long as you schedule it on a day when you are free of to-dos and can fully immerse yourself in the experience. Depending on the spa, a typical day package might involve a massage, a facial, a light lunch, access to a sauna or aromatic steam room, a manicure, and pedicure. You'll leave the spa after a few hours feeling relaxed and refreshed.

If you can't afford a spa day, create your own with a friend, family member, or lover. Set up your bedroom with candles, put in a relaxing CD or playlist, and cover your bed with a super soft towel. Pick up a bottle of unscented massage oil or a massage oil that has the essence of lavender, rose, jojoba, or another relaxing scent. Have the person receiving the massage lie down on the bed, put some oil in your hands to warm it up, and start working on your partner (or friend). Make sure to go slowly and cover all the parts of the body that the other person is comfortable with you massaging. After you're finished and your partner (or spa buddy) has taken a few moments to enjoy the feeling of their body post-massage, switch places. If you want to really make it feel like a spa, have some cucumber slices and other items on hand to make homemade facial masks, and consider giving each other manis and pedis. Men can enjoy those as well, even if they opt for no polish.

"In everyone's life, at some time, our inner fire goes out. It is then burst into flame by an encounter with another human being. We should all be thankful for those people who rekindle the inner spirit."

—Albert Schweitzer

Try a Little Friend Therapy

Friend therapy is simple: Let your friends help you manage your stress! Research shows that people without social networks and friends often feel lonely, but often won't admit it. If you don't have a ready-to-go group of friends or have lost touch with yours, one of the easiest ways to make friends is to join something. Take a class, join a club, attend a church, find a support group. You might need to try a few different things before you meet people you can really relate to, but if you keep trying, you'll do it.

Friend therapy isn't complicated. All it entails is human contact—not cyber-contact (although that's better than no contact). Phone contact can be helpful, but nothing beats the real thing. Just being with another person—talking (even if it's not about your problems), having fun, taking a break from the daily routine—is a great way to relax, raise your self-esteem, and have the chance to be there for somebody else, too. You don't have to do anything in particular with your friends to make it friend therapy. You just have to get a social life.

AFTERWORD

"We learn by practice. Whether it means to learn to dance by practicing dancing or to learn to live by practicing living, the principles are the same. . . . One becomes in some area an athlete of God."

—Martha Graham

Assess Your Health Success

Now that the year's at its end, this is a great time to review your progress on all fronts. One of the best ways to see how far you've come and to plot changes for the upcoming year is to spend a few minutes assessing your progress. Answer the following questions:

- Have you improved your diet? Have you cut way back on saturated fats, while increasing good fats? Have you added more fruits and vegetables? Are you making sure you are eating vitamin-rich foods?
- Are your muscles stronger than they were a year ago? Are you able to lift heavier weights, or increase your reps? Have you noticed an improved ability to perform everyday tasks?
- Are you eating foods that nourish your brain? Do you regularly do activities that will keep your brain supple? Do you challenge your brain? Do you make sure you get thirty minutes of exercise daily to keep your brain functioning at peak capacity?
- Have you kept abreast with the increasing difficulty and duration of the exercise programs offered in this book? Do your regularly push yourself just a little harder? Are you ready to add a more strenuous regime, such as running three times a week?
- Have you added yoga (or a similar routine, such as Tai Chi) to your weekly workouts? Do you consciously execute the types of stretches that will facilitate flexibility? Do you alternate workouts to focus on various sets of muscles (shoulders and arms one day; buttocks and legs the next)?

- Do you make time for recreational activities? Do you make sure that your recreational activities are ones that give your body a workout? Do you have a hobby that you do regularly? Have you cut back on time spent watching TV?
- Do you make time to rest? Have you tried meditation? Do you have rituals that nourish your soul? Have you grown to know yourself — and what pleases you — better? Are you able to quiet your mind and truly relax?

In answering these questions, you may be pleasantly surprised to discover how far you really have come, and what a difference working toward the healthiest you ever has made in your overall health and happiness. If you fell short, simply start the new year by starting over; if you've done fairly well, go back and focus on the activities that you didn't adopt; if you've done really well, keep up your program, coming up with your own ideas for ways to bolster your progress.

To all, major congratulations on valuing yourself enough to buy this book and spend the time to institute changes that will make a huge difference in your life.

INDEX

Eagle pose, 248
Elliptical trainers, 304
Energy drinks, 96
Ergometers, 290
Essential oils, 171

Farmer's markets, 170
Fartlek, 197
Fats, dietary, 58, 74, 88, 103, 136, 210
Fiber, 79, 136
Fish, 65, 81
Fish oil capsules, 117
Flaxseed oil, 88
Food diaries, 1
Friends, 239, 371
Front kick-back kick combination, 345
Fruits, 93

Gardens, 127, 149
Garlic, 244
Ginkgo biloba, 246
Golf, 62
Grains, whole vs. refined, 51
Gratitude, expressing, 185
Green Bloody Mary, 131
Greens, leafy, 107
Green soup, 330
Green tea, 337
Gym, joining, 23

Habitat for Humanity, 242
Hand-weights, 6
Heart rate monitors, 108
Herbs, 127, 164, 365
High knee skip, 245
Hiking, 285
Himalayas, trekking, 349
Hips, range and flexibility improvement, 291
Hobbies, 105, 335
Hops, 329
Horseback riding, 235
Hummus, 322
Hunger, helping to relieve, 336
Hydration, 96, 301

Indigestion relief, 78
Injuries, minimizing, 316
Intensity of workout, increasing, 189
Interval training, 333
Iron-rich foods, 358

Jumping jacks (in the pool), 268
Jumping lunges, 287

Kale, 258
Karvonen formula, 18
Kettle bell swing (double-arm swing), 309
Kickboxing, 356
Kicks, 166

Lateral pushes, 252
Lavender, 14, 99
Lectures, attending, 45
Leg exercises, 126, 261, 304
Leg extensions, 104
Legs-up-the-wall pose, 255
Lemon balm extract, 157
Low-level activities, 368
Lunge pose, 291
Lunges, 195, 287

Magnesium, 253
Mantras, 300, 357
Marathons, avoiding, 68
Massage, 21, 140, 221, 305
Media, 192
Meditation, 38, 92, 153, 178, 214, 243, 300, 357
Memory, 102, 367
Mercury in fish, 81
Metabolism boosting, 40, 43
Metabolism calculators, 8
Micro-plants, 286
Models (airplane, train, ship), 328
Moderate activity, 41
Motivation, 168
Mountain pose, 234
Movies, funny, 53
Music, 70, 134

ABOUT THE AUTHORS

Meera Lester is the author of more than two dozen books, including *365 Ways to Live the Law of Attraction* and *The Everything® Law of Attraction Book*. She lives in San Jose, CA.

Murdoc Khaleghi, MD, author of *The Everything® Low Cholesterol Book, 2nd Edition*, is an emergency physician attending in Massachusetts. After studying biomedical engineering and medicine at the University of California, San Diego, he trained in emergency medicine through Tufts University. Dr. Khaleghi has earned numerous research fellowships from institutions such as the American Heart Association, the National Institutes of Health, the Howard Hughes Medical Institute, and Stein Institute for Research on Aging, which he has used to perform research on topics ranging from cardiovascular disorders to the benefits of cholesterol-lowering drugs.

Susan Reynolds has a BA in psychology and is the owner and founder of Literary Cottage, a literary consulting firm based in Boston, through which she coaches other writers in pursuit of happiness through publishing. She co-authored *Train Your Brain to Get Happy* and *Train Your Brain to Get Rich*, and writes a blog entitled "Prime Your Gray Cells" on Psychologytoday.com. She lives in Boston, MA.

Brett Aved is a personal trainer located in Napa, California. Aved has been an athlete and fitness enthusiast for more than fifteen years and has trained in various capacities, including weightlifting, mixed martial arts, and Krav Maga. He believes in overall fitness achieved through various methods, with an individualized focus on each client's nutrition needs, physical capabilities, and drive.